Taboo Secrets of Pregnancy

A Guide to Life with a Belly

By Michelle Smith, M.S., SLP

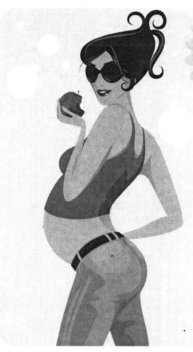

"The Inside Scoop on being Pregnant!"

Library of Congress Cataloging-in-Publication Data has been applied for.

ISBN-13: 978-1-45366-716-3 • ISBN-10: 1-45366-716-4

Cover design, interior, illustrations, and photos by Chris Smith.

Printed and bound in the United States of America

First Edition

Note to Readers: This book is intended for entertainment and informational purposes only and does not replace the advice of medical professionals. Readers should consult their obstetrician or other trained medical experts before acting on any of the information in this book.

With greatest joy, we are blessed to announce the arrival of our little bundle of "Hope".

Miss Evelyn "Wee Baby" ...welcome to the family!

Contents

Acknowledgements

To Leslie Fossen: HO-ly cow, girl. Your caliber of wit and smarts puts us mere mortals to absolute shame. Endless thanks, oh-ye-goddess of editing, for sweeping in and saving my batooty! I feel so privileged and grateful for your input, contribution to content, and pregnant mommy eyes fixing my prose. How lucky does one get?!

To Monica, for your boost to the ego. Thank you for your support on this potty-mouth project and for laughing your butt off in all the right places.

To my Poker Mommies, for your laughter, insight, lack of sympathy and scandalous stories!

To Amy, for being so entertaining and letting me splatter your outrageous antics all over my books. For two people who are absolutely no fun, we sure do have a lot of fun! Three cheers for expensive chocolate!

To Miss Sas-a-Fras Wee, for gracing me with such misery and giving me something to write about! I adore your precious hugs and Sweet Wee's Sweet Tea. Love you, Weesa.

To Poppy and Mimi: To answer your question, "YEESSS!" I am finally finished working on this book! Thank you for the frequent interruptions and hugs. I love you, babies!

To Chris: Woohoo! Need I say more? High five, honey!

Introduction: Shell-Shock

Yea! We're making a baby! Cool!

And then...reality sets in. Crap. You know, I really feel like crap! Great balls of fire, this was supposed to be all fun and mushy and happy! What the (bleep!) is happening to me, and by the way, get me some dadgum cheese-fries NOW!

Okay, so there are exceptions to the rule, but for many of us down-to-earth gals, being pregnant is no cake walk. In fact, it's not even a cupcake or junior sundae. More like a fried fish sandwich; stinky and ugly, but delicious all the same.

Yes, I've actually met a couple of women who gush how they've never felt better and how they can't wait to do it again (give me a rotten tomato and I will throw), but for the most part, pregnancy is a journey into seriously foreign and freaky territory.

There are certainly a few good books on pregnancy and childbirth, but 99% of them are written to provide technical information. Nothing wrong with this of course, but it would be a great relief to those of you new to the process to get some completely frank and practical advice as well. Not only will I be disgustingly candid on the taboo stuff your doctor and mother seem to gloss over, but there is another little twist to this book you might find comforting:

I'm pregnant!

I just found out that my third child is on the way. Having run this race twice before, I still could have written a witty book on the realities of pregnancy without actually being in the family way, but the fact of the matter is that when you are pregnant, reality is different. Mother Nature makes you forget quickly, and writing a book on pregnancy when (a) you aren't going through it, or (b) never have and never will – eh, hem....male authors – just isn't the same.

Sorry Mr. Medical Guys, but there is a certain bonding element missing when the blessed event will never riddle <u>your</u> body with gas and burps and farts, the likes of which would bring down an elephant. (HOW does that much air get in my body?! Crimony!) Seriously, no offense. I'm sure your point of view has great irrational-yelling-wife-or-patient observations, but the hormonal upheaval just isn't punching you in quite the same way. Nor is it punching those of you for which pregnancy is a happy, distant memory. For all I know, you could have serious nature-induced-brain-washed-amnesia by now, and you've blissfully forgotten all the heebie-jeebie disgusting goo and gas and blood and just general ick that goes along with being preggers.

If you haven't already, you will come to find out that pregnant women gravitate toward each other. You can be in a grocery store or mall and your hormonal radar will kick in high gear if another pregnant woman is within 100 yards. Yoohoo, hello! Hey girlfriend! Instinctively drawn to each other, you have no qualms immediately opening up on bouts of nausea, heartburn, and leaky nipples. A complete stranger becomes immediate "sis-ta!"

Here's where I step in. This book is in no way a technical or medical guide, and I am no doctor, midwife, or physician's assistant. I'm simply a very honest chic who has been down this road a couple of times and putting on my running shoes again. This book is the necessary supplement to your basic medical reference on pregnancy and will fill in the gaps where those boring books won't tread. I won't drone on and on about the technical stuff, because you already know all that. But if you want a heart-to-heart on the realities of pregnancy, grab a blanket and cup of tea (decaf!) and sit right down with me, girly.

As you read, feel certain I am going through the stages I write about. While I will try to maintain a modicum of respectable language, I'm racing down a hormonal hill, girlfriend. Decency might take a hike, so be prepared and please forgive if I offend any delicate sensibilities! Outspoken on a good day, I'm thinking the potty mouth sailor will take over once we hit the second trimester. Either way, I refuse to sugarcoat truths or lie about how big our butts will get. We will go through this hormonal adventure together, holding our heads high, puking our guts out, and commiserating in detail. I am here to be your friend and guide, and intend to get you through these next nine months with confidence, laughter, and empathy. If you pee in your pants on my account, great! That's what true friends are for.

Okay. Now that I've wiped those dadgum hormonal tears, let our journey begin...

Chapter One: Let the Fun Begin!

So. You've either heard the word from your doctor or you've peed on that stick and watched in eager anticipation for the little pink line (or blue line, or plus sign, or whatever the heck it is) to appear. Congratulations! Doubt may constantly linger because you can't believe you're really pregnant, but believe me, honey, you are.

If you're just dying to know that your symptoms are real, let's run down the basics and get you convinced that you are, in fact, wonderfully knocked up. You'll soon be sporting granny panties and loving it! (You think I lie, but oh honey, are you in for it!)

1. The Obvious: A Missed Period. Technically, you are supposed to start your period two weeks after you ovulate, but who the dickens knows when that is? If your body isn't very cooperative with the cycle business, just count four weeks from the first day of your last period. You should have another period somewhere in that general vicinity. If you haven't started within about 7-10 days from that date, go ahead and take a pregnancy test. However, you and I both know you will just DIE if you have to wait 7-10 days, so grab one of those super-early tests and give it a whirl. You may end up flushing a lot of money down the toilet in your fervent need to know <u>right now</u>, but for goodness sake! It's a little babino we're talking about, here! You go for it, girl.

While we're on the subject, to most women, the prospect of having no periods for nine months is so inviting that getting pregnant and caring for a child for the next eighteen years is a very small price to pay. However, don't get too worked up. In fact, be prepared to feel royally gypped with all the disgusting goo coming out of our supposedly period-free space. Keep those pantiliners handy and don't panic over the frequent goopy rushes down there. You'll probably high-tail it to the bathroom in a frenzy of worry that you're bleeding ("I know it! This is it. It's blood this time!") when in fact, it's just another one of Mother Nature's cruel tricks. With as much mucus, blood, and slime that squirts

5

out when you actually have the kid, you would think the ol' uterus packs it away like a squirrel preparing for winter, but no. There's a constant flood of viscous-alien-like-yuck navigating your hoochy-hoo, making you nuts. GROSS!

2. *A Positive Pregnancy Test.* Oh, that little stick! For some reason, first-timers seem to think these tests can have all kinds of faults and refuse to believe the accuracy. The truth is, I haven't met a woman yet who has had a false positive. If the test says you're pregnant, assume you are.

Sometimes that little line will be very faint, but that's still a positive. It just means that there isn't a ton of the HCG hormone (one of those things you already know about) in your body. If you get a faint line, you've probably tested a little early and will get a darker line if you wait a few days and test again. Either way, positive is positive. And for those of us who scream at those dang lines, "Is it there? Is it not there? What the hell is this stick doing?!" - those smart little scientists in lab coats have designed sticks that say "pregnant" or "not pregnant." I for one am thrilled, since it's taken me three pregnancies to get this test thing down pat.

3. *Fatigue.* Mama Jama! The first trimester brings monstrous changes to your body – mainly, making the placenta. Just brushing your teeth feels like hiking Everest. It takes a colossal amount of effort for your body to get through this initial stage, and this freakish tired is normal, girlfriend. Your energy should pick up once the placenta is done cooking. (Then it flattens again and you'll feel like dying, but we'll get to that later.)

4. *"Stomach" Problems: Kill me, Float me, and Get-it-Out!* Indigestion, gas, bloating, and constipation. Ooooh, love it! Cola burns a hole in your throat, and pizza nearly keels you over; just one more sign that a certain little someone is giving you the fetus version of "up yours!" Our food choices seem to piss the little tyke off daily. If he happens to actually like your culinary selection, you may get the opposite treatment, and the kid won't let you get rid of it. And thus you are initiated into the Get-This-Shit-Out-of-Me Constipation Club. Overall, pregnancy can wreak some serious havoc on your bowels and digestive system, so be prepared for some major adjustments if you want things to run anywhere close to happy. Your poor little butt will thank you.

5. *Distraction.* Mercy alive! Can we just freaking think?! Ummm...nope. With gestating hot on the brain, you lose all ability to concentrate, and that's that. Forget trying to figure it out. You may find yourself driving down the road and slamming on the brakes because you're gazing at the clouds instead of the Mack truck three feet in front of you. Or hubby has to ask eight times what movie you want to watch as you give him a glassy-eyed stare. Huh? You say something?

6. *Sore "Girls".* Ah yes, those poor, poor boobs. They swell and ache (and swear and cuss) so bad that lightly hugging a family friend will make you wince or cry out in agony, "Aahhh, ouch! My boobs!" Yes, you will get a few stares of disbelief, but the party crushing your tender knockers is not pregnant, so they cannot possibly understand your pain. So look out, make way, and handle with care! Pregnant boobs, coming through!

7. *Need to Pee, Please!* Once the little interloper is growing in your belly, the first thing you'll want to do is pee. Girl, I'm fully aware that you may have just peed on a stick or in a cup, but you'll need to go again. I have no idea why your body thinks it needs to pee so much, but such is life. And when you've got to pee, you have got to PEE. Little old ladies better get the heck out of the way, lest they land on the floor.

8. *Ouufff! (Clumsiness):* Butter fingers and big feet while pregnant is just SO delightful. Hells bells, I drop the milk while pouring, the spoon while eating, the brush while brushing, and shatter about one glass per week all over my kitchen floor. I trip on carpet, run into walls, drop my keys, fall off the bed, and whack my hip on the corner of my counters (I WILL saw those damn things off!) My hubby, who thinks this is all quite hilarious, gets a slew of profanities and hairy eyeballs daily, as I'm feeling quite sorry for myself and not in the mood to be laughed at.

I've known women who have stumbled over curbs and landed on their butts, or tripped on nothing at all and landed flat on their faces. This is inevitable in the life of the pregnant woman, as (a) you're so dizzy that no object of focus will sit still, much less the floor, and (b) once your belly is big enough to enter a room before you do, balance simply takes a hike.

9. *I'm an Emotional Train Wreck!* Around the time you find out you're pregnant, your hormones – oh hell, they just dive off a cliff, girlfriend. Welcome to the next eight months. Thrilled and happy as a puppy one minute, mean and hissy as a pit viper the next. Yep, you've arrived. Never in your life would you have suspected you could so easily cry during a tire commercial. Or you can be happily playing with your children at the park, then boom! It takes every ounce of your being not to kick the little heathen who beats your child to the swings. Rotten little toot-faced brat!

In addition to bursts of fury, you will be overwhelmed, full of anticipation, excitement, and worry. A few of you lucky gals are as laid back as a gummy worm on a beach, but the rest of us fret and agonize over every little pregnant detail. We worry about the baby. We worry about how fat we'll get, whose advice we should actually listen to, the medication we took (damnit!), or that glass of wine before we knew. If you're sick, you worry. If you're not, you worry. Am I progressing? Is the baby growing? Why don't I feel different? Why do I feel so bad?

Now, the thing about worrying is that it does you absolutely no good. I can't actually tout that my little brain doesn't get worked up over nothing, even the third time around, but I do arm myself with a little bit of knowledge and comfort. I have finally learned that all I can do is take care of myself. Take your vitamins, eat right, exercise as your doctor permits, don't smoke, and don't take drugs. Beyond that, *let it go.*

My best friend Amy happens to be one of the smartest cookies I know. Yet she still went into brain-lock when she got pregnant, putting herself into a frenzy over -get this- toxoplasmosis. For those of you unfamiliar, toxoplasmosis is one of those bugs you need to stay away from when you're gestating. One of the ways it's transmitted is through cat feces, and the way to keep it at bay is to let someone else clean the litter box while you're pregnant. Make sure they thoroughly clean their hands after scooping the poop, and you'll be fine.

Since Amy and I both happen to be speech therapists, we're a bit more familiar with the virus than most people, because it can cause neurological damage in children. But knowing exactly what toxoplasmosis does and where it comes from was of no comfort to Amy. She was agonizing - not over the fact that she actually had three cats and possibly cleaned the box before she knew she was pregnant - but because she had been "exposed" to farm cats when she was a little girl. She'd played with the little mongrels nearly twenty years ago, and was now worried that she'd contracted the disease back then and never knew it.

It took me half a freaking day to calm the woman down and convince her to get over it. In order for the virus to harm your fetus, you have to actually contract it *while* you are pregnant. Now, did Amy listen to me on this point? Nope. Did she already *know* this point? Of course. So was I wasting my breath and speaking to an irrational person? Yes! It took some serious bribes of pickled asparagus and cheesecake to get her focused on something else.

Nonsense like this is useless to worry about. But it will happen, no matter how down-to-earth and practical you are. Amy worried herself to death over toxoplasmosis, yet five months later got a tongue lashing from her doctor because she showed up for her check-up reeking of bleach. She'd been merrily cleaning bathrooms all day and didn't think twice about the nasty chemical burning a hole in her nose. Yowza! There's a preggy brain for ya!

Speaking of Amy, now is a good time to introduce you to the Poker Mommies. Amy introduced me to this nifty group of women, and it was instant bonding from the moment we bit into our dinner tacos (watching most of the ingredients fall onto our lactating breasts). We now get together once a month for the legendary "Poker Night." We don't actually *play* poker (although Teresa keeps bringing chips in high hopes of a good gamble), but it started out as a poker group, so the name stuck. We are a tight knit group of gals who each have a kid or two, and heavens alive, they just keep coming. Someone is always pregnant or postpartum (our record is four preggos at once), so you can imagine the food. Fried pickles, hot wings, taco soup, and Thai meet the needs of many on any given night, although the unfortunate host-husband may feel a strong need to barf.

The Poker Mommies are my team of consultants, dear friends, and fun buddies. We laugh, cry, gripe, commiserate, and stuff our faces together. Any time I am researching a book or have some oddball question, I automatically consult the group for a balanced opinion. We've been through it all, and being a rather honest group of ladies, they certainly won't beat around the bush about what it's really like to be pregnant. You will find that I refer to my little posse often, as their stories are rich with humor, insight, and sometimes quite wonderful scandal.

Bendy Plans Are Good Plans

Being the great researching mom-to-be that you are, of course you will rush right out and get a bundle of technical pregnancy guides to get a second, third, and fourth opinion on everything related to gestating and child rearing. Well and good, as you will probably refer to all of your books often. However, having a library of them myself, I will give you fair warning. When you get yourself a text for information on tests, procedures, and general physical changes, be very wary. Try to find one that presents a neutral point of view, because medical factoids or not, really honey, they are chock full of the author's opinion. How-to books and guides are written with a slant – no big secret – but when newly preggers, you have entered a totally new world. Don't take books you read as gospel. In reality, you have lots of options. If an author suggests, pushes, persuades, or cajoles you to do any of the following, he/she may be a tad biased to one extreme or the other:

- Encourages natural childbirth at home because the author herself has cranked out about ten kids that way, and, gosh, it's a beautiful and relatively pain-free experience.

- Scares you into thinking a medical doctor is the only feasible option since your birthing parts will surely need to be sewn up like a ripped seam.

- Advises you breastfeed until your child is old enough to suggest that it's time to move on to a cup.

- Tells you it's cruel to make your child sleep anywhere but with you until the kid comes into the bedroom one day, tosses the car keys on the dresser, and says, "You know, I've got a job now, so I think I'll go out and buy myself a bed."

Decisions you make during pregnancy and child rearing should be yours. Take everything you read with a grain of salt, and don't let anyone push or guilt you into doing something you are not comfortable with. Just keep an open mind when it comes to prenatal care and childbirth because the blessed event doesn't always go as planned. Ultimately, this is your body, your pregnancy, and your path to follow. Choose a plan A and choose a plan B. Then reserve the right to change your dadgum mind as you please.

Think Again, Girl: Here's the Poker Group's first piece of advice: when it comes to gestating, take any and all preconceived notions about what you think it's like to be pregnant, and chuck them out the window. Pregnancy and childbirth have a tendency to throw you a few loops, so try to keep an open mind and not get your heart set on how you're supposed to feel, act, or look. It's well and good to have a plan, but don't set your expectations too high. If things fall short, those hysterical hormones will kick to life, and you might start breaking all your china.

Being pregnant is a roller coaster ride; pretty much guaranteed to be bumpy but also quite thrilling. When you go into it prepared for the unexpected, you're much better off. I know a few people who were dead set on having their babies a certain way, then heartbroken when complications arose, forcing them to abandon their idea of a perfect birthing experience. You need to keep focused on your main goal – a healthy baby.

No matter what your plan, whether you are determined to have a natural or pain-free birth, medication or no medication, breastfeeding or no breastfeeding, just keep your options open. Allow yourself the liberty to change your mind on what you've decided, and try to avoid a laser focus on doing one thing versus the other. There is no reason to feel guilty for deciding you want an epidural at the last minute. There is also no reason to be pushed into *getting* an epidural if you make a last minute choice to go ahead without it. If it's your first baby, you absolutely will not know how labor will affect you and how you will want to proceed until you're there. Have a plan, but keep it flexible, and allow for contingencies.

Choosing a Doc to Poop On

With your basic plan comes a basic decision: who do you want to deliver this baby and how do you want to do it? A doctor or midwife? Hospital or not? Again, you may have to make adjustments should any complications arise, but go ahead and pick the method and expert you think will suit you. Just remember, you've got to be comfortable with them. You're building a very personal relationship with someone who will get to know your naked parts on a first name basis, end up covered in your bodily fluids (and solids), and ask you questions you'd prefer not to reveal to your dog.

And here's another bummer: if you chose a doctor in a group practice, you might be forced to rotate through each one toward the end of your prenatal appointments. Think about it. You'll get stuck with whoever is on call during your labor. Period. End of story. That's the dude (or chick) who will deliver your baby. So sometimes they'll rotate your appointments - and have yet another person stick their hand up your peanut. This way you can meet each doctor and not be freaked out when you're spread eagle in Labor & Delivery, about to start pushing. In floats a scrub garbed stranger getting right to business, rubbing and stretching the door of your hoo-hoo in preparation for birth. Hello, sir! Nice to meet you and your hands all over my privates!

Now, sometimes you are stuck because you need a specialist for a high-risk pregnancy, but you can still have the support of a midwife if you'd like. Many doctors work in conjunction with midwife services. If so, jump on it. If not, see if your specialist can recommend some support groups or childbirth classes geared toward your specific needs. It can be lonely and downright depressing for pregnancy or childbirth to become a serious and frightful event. Do your best to connect with other women who are going through the same thing or have been there.

For a normal ol' run-of-the-mill pregnancy, keep an open mind about having a doctor on hand if you want a natural childbirth with a midwife. Give yourself latitude to change your mind about pain medication because you never know what labor and birth will be like. Of my two friends who insisted on natural births, one ended up being so exhausted that she had to have an epidural simply so she could rest for a couple hours before pushing. The other one needed surgery, and the baby ended up in the Neonatal Intensive Care Unit for months.

On the other side, I also have a sister who had three natural births at home and was determined to have baby number four with a midwife, at a hospital, with an epidural. It turned out that my nephew was five weeks early and practically fell out. This left my sister in unwanted agony with a complete stranger rushing in the hospital room just in time to catch the baby like a football. My sister did end up getting the epidural she so desperately wanted, but she either got it too late or it just didn't "take", giving her no relief from the pain. Not only that, but she got stuck with an insensitive cad delivering her child. He was pulling and tugging and slicing and dicing like she was a piece of meat instead of a woman with pain receptors in high gear.

I share all this not to scare you, but simply to convince you to prepare for unforeseen events. In all likelihood, your birth will be a wonderful experience. It might have a few hiccups, but if you prepare and arm yourself with research and knowledge, the amazing event should run smoothly. Then there you'll be, pleased as punch when that gorgeous baby is placed in your arms!

All in all, these are just a few of the wonders, problems, and questions you will experience when you first find out you're pregnant. It's all new, crazy, and wonderful. Enjoy those first few weeks of basking in the knowledge of growing a tiny life inside you. Walk around smiling, rubbing your belly, whatever you want. Take pleasure in it now because your body is slowly being taken over, and you may soon be confused and fervently ticked at Mother Nature's wild ride. Have fun!

Chapter Two: Hey! Who Stole My Body?

Once you hit about four to five weeks of gestation, your brow may begin to furrow as you wake up one morning feeling "different." Hmmm…wonder what that could be? Twelve seconds later, you fly to the bathroom and hurl your last meal in agony.

There is some major construction going on in your uterus, and for some reason, it seems to affect every single aspect of your physical and emotional life. How such a tiny creature can cause such angst, I'm sure I don't know. But no one said it would be easy! (At least not to my face. The first time I actually meet a bozo like that, they're getting the back of my pregnant hand.) The changes your body will endure are shocking, to be sure, but equally thrilling and awe-inspiring.

Pukeyland, USA

Just a Little Pukey (Regular Ol' Nausea): Okay, so maybe morning sickness isn't exactly thrilling and awe-inspiring. And let's take a moment to discuss this stupidly loose term. Just WHO the hell made up the "morning" part? Morning, my butt! It's all the time! Dear God, pul-eze just let me throw up so I can be happy and hungry again!

Nausea – or even the thought of it, is so "oh-my-gosh, I'm really pregnant" and quite nifty in the beginning, but great merciful goose, it gets old quick. A bewildering conundrum, you will often find yourself fluctuating between starving and wanting to puke. The wonder of it all is that nothing seems to help. Puking doesn't always make you feel *less* like puking, and eating doesn't always remedy the insane hunger. Sometimes you will eat and immediately run to the can to toss your cookies. And you would think that getting rid of the offending food would lessen the intense anger that your stomach obviously feels toward you, but no. You can throw up every ounce of sustenance you've had for 24 hours, and your stomach will still be pissed off, forcing you to lie in bed, unable to move. Or worse, the old tum-tum continues to punish your glowing-pregnant self, making you dry heave until you're coughing up bile.

The thing about nausea is this: if you have the mild ickiness that accompanies many pregnancies, all the remedies you find in your medical texts and the peachy advice from others will get you through just fine. With my first two pregnancies, about ten crackers and half a bottle of Emetrol sailed me through with only a few moments of, "Uuuhhh. I don't feel so good." This third time around, however, all that cracker-action was smoke up my fanny for all the good it did – but we'll get to that.

For your run-of-the-mill nausea, try all the conventional "food" methods. One possible reason for the nausea is that your hormones are on overdrive trying to get that little critter and his placenta formed. Your blood sugar is completely out of whack and will fall without frequent small meals. When it falls, you get queasy, shaky, irritable, and just generally crazed. If you eat often, *before* you get hungry, you can head off a good deal of this blood sugar nonsense. Carey, one of my pregnant Poker Mommies, reports that as long as she's chewing, she's good.

Eat foods that don't make you gag, and shoot for a balance of dairy, protein, fruits, vegetables, and grains. It's not always doable, so don't sweat it. Just eat what you feel you can get down at the moment, and avoid greasy, fatty, highly seasoned or spicy foods. If 3-alarm chili sounds great for dinner, go for it, but don't call me crying when you're up all night in stomach-hell.

You've all read the basic books and know those pregnancy diets, so I won't go into huge detail here. Suffice it to say that if you stick to rather bland, naturally sweet foods, you're more likely to keep the nausea monster at bay. Believe me, I know how difficult it is to eat healthy when you feel like crap on a stick, but it's worth a try.

Puke-a-Rama! (Severe Nausea): Now, most pregnancy books will gloss over a term called *hyperemesis gravidarum*, and frankly, it's a crying shame. The reason being is that most women don't actually suffer from this extreme form of nausea and vomiting, so I guess it doesn't behoove writers to bother with it. However, having had a peek down this particularly retched trail, I've found that if you do suffer from it, this is what happens: you're left to feel like you should be feeling better if you just follow all the "advice" on nausea, and if you don't feel better, something is wrong with you. After fighting the crackers, dried fruit, rice cakes, plenty of fluids, breads, cheese, nuts, applesauce, ginger tea, broths, blah, blah, blah, and no relief is in sight, you begin to wonder if you're all alone and completely misunderstood by the rest of the world.

I have spent my entire first trimester trying to choke down all the appropriate bland foods when, where, and how I'm supposed to. But after bawling my eyes out trying to gag down two bites of bran muffin and some milk, I realized things were a bit different this time around. So, with the advice of my doctor, I gave other methods a go: changing vitamins, putting sea bands on my wrists (what the hell ARE those things??), taking a vitamin regimen of 50mg B6, ½ a Unisom before bed (supposedly to help cut morning nausea and help you sleep), Emetrol, and replacing some of my water intake with something that had some sugar and flavor, like Sprite or Gatorade. Surprisingly, plain water sometimes makes things worse - a testament you may actually hear from women who end up dehydrated in the ER because they just can't swallow the stuff.

When all medical advice and well-intentioned suggestions from friends and family still left me bed bound, unable to care for my children, unable to perform basic daily tasks, and crying myself to sleep, I had my epiphany. I realized that if something could not be done, I was going to perish – taking my poor innocent fetus right along with me. Luckily, I had to drag my sorry self into the doctor one particularly bad morning to pick up some vitamins from the OB nurse. She took one look at me, left the room, and came back with a sample of a little pill that would change everything.

Now, I am absolutely the tree-hugging kind of person who loathes taking medicine. Even in a non-pregnant state, anything stronger than Tylenol gets a growl of distain. So. Here's the thing. Yes, I HATE the idea of possibly harming my baby by taking any form of medication that isn't absolutely necessary. But for me, it was absolutely necessary.

First of all, I rationalized that there are plenty of perfectly safe drugs to take while pregnant. While we are sometimes hesitant to actually believe the medical community on this one, there is a point of concession. I would never tell you what to do, girlfriend, but personally, I had to roll over and accept the fact that my doctor knows the research a little better than your average, hormonally crazed and desperately ill pregnant woman (me).

Second, there are some people who are too sick to function or get enough calories, and seriously need the help. *You* may be able to bravely suffer through the horrible ordeal, but your *baby* needs some nutrition and sustenance. If you aren't getting enough food and fluids to keep yourself going, what makes you think your baby is getting enough to do all that rapid growing?

So, while my "magic" (and horrifically expensive) anti-nausea prescription pill didn't actually fix my problems completely, it certainly kept me going enough that I could, at the very least, eat a little more and get some sleep. For the most part, I was able to stretch out the dosage from two pills per day to one pill every other day, so I felt a little better about not over medicating my child. However, the nausea was still so severe that I had to stop taking my prenatal vitamins, and my doctor urged me to take more medicine so I could get back on the vitamins and gain some weight. I didn't follow the advice partly because of my fear of drugs and partly because of the horrid side effect this particular medication had on me.

One word: shit. No wait – HARD shit. Coal in your gut. Rocks. Tree trunks. Yeah, that's better! Let's just rename this medication "Can't Shit but Helps with Nausea." Sweet mother of mercy, I'm already in the Can't Crap Club! Will no one throw me a bone? Wonderfully safe drug or not, Captain Weenie here had to battle daily with a gallon of prune juice, a very large bottle of Metamucil tablets, and every green and fiberous food I could manage to choke down. It eventually worked, although not without some severe cramping, more than a few tears, and a very sore butt.

Bottom line, if you need the help – it's okay. Just talk to your doctor about options, and weigh the risks. I've now known four women diagnosed with hyperemesis gravidarum, each of whom had to be on medication, and each of whom had wonderfully healthy babies. In fact, one of them was so sick that her second pregnancy landed her in the ICU with a feeding tube and failing kidneys. She eventually had to alternate four different medications every two hours. The medications didn't relieve the nausea, but they did keep her from puking ten times an hour.

Stomach Problems & "Fartle"

It never fails to astonish when a seasoned pregger picks up an arbitrary pregnancy guide and reads a lame, Barbie-like, chipper comment, "You may be feeling slightly bloated and gassy." HELL-O!! Slightly bloated and gassy?! How about "I'm farting so much that my husband calls me 'Oh Ye Gaseous One' and the bloating is more along the lines of exploding?" There. Much more realistic.

Speaking of realistic, let's discuss childbirth classes. Forget the actual fear of birth. Just getting through the hour-long class can be a gassy, belchy, wind-blowing nightmare if you happen to get the right group of unfortunately afflicted women. Out pops a chorus of farts followed closely by smothered laughter from fathers-to-be as the mommies land their big bellies down on the floor (a feat in and of itself). Breathing exercises are sure to elicit more music. And as soon as the pushing practice begins, stifle your snicker or you will be viciously kicked out by several unhappy mamas and one ticked-off instructor.

The gas of pregnancy is probably most uncomfortable in the first trimester, but even as the intense bloating fades, the amount of air coming out of your body is shocking. Thus, the "fartle" (fart+startle). You know how a dog will toot, then spin his head around, raise his ears, and stare at his butt in wonder? Yep. That's what it's like. You can be walking down a hallway farting so much that it seems to scoot you along like a propulsion engine. What the...??? Or you can be in your car belting out a song with Celine Dion, and all of a sudden you burp so loudly that (a) you quickly assess how many other drivers saw your mouth open for that long, and (b) you startle yourself into missing a turn. I don't know how many times I've been in my car on the way to church or a meeting, belched out a big one, then started chanting, "You can't do that in public, you can't do that in public!"

So, how to avoid the gassy-gal syndrome? Hmmm. Well, your basic eat-healthy-pregnancy-diet should help, but ask your doctor about leaning on the over-the-counter methods like Gas-X or Mylicon. Steer clear of carbonated beverages (duh), and of course, those wonderful buffalo wings and other spicy and processed foods (rats!).

If I sound rather unenthusiastic on this, it's actually because of my tendency to lean toward Mother Nature. I'm not convinced that anything you do will make a dramatic difference. I think She will make and release gas when She feels like it, and avoiding gas-producing foods can only help lessen the tooting, not ax it. Eating very nearly like a rabbit, your gas-producing-wonder of a belly could still refuse to notice or care. When that happens, just rustle your feet or make some noise and hope and pray that no one hears. If you're lucky enough to be home on a bad day, relief may be in sight if you can take a nice long visit to the toilet. Squeeze in a few Olympic-worthy belches while you're at it.

Head & Nose Blues

Well, Hello Headache! (Where's the Tylenol?!) Just as those gestating hormones turn the rest of your bodily functions into matters of weird science, they'll give your head a spin too – and you are in fine company. Whether it's from hormones, food odors, allergies, blood sugar, fatigue, stress, or voodoo, headaches tend to multiply and intensify during pregnancy.

The first thing you need to do is check your diet. It's possible that many of your headaches could be directly due to the food you're eating. Caffeine and chocolate are the obvious culprits, but there could be other little offenders lurking about. Green tea was my bad guy – which sucks because it's supposed to be good for you, but oh well. If your head starts hurting after you eat, keep a log of the meals. Find out which foods are bothersome and nix them. It could save you a lot of time and, um, headaches.

Other ways to evade the pesky head pain is to get enough rest, avoid stress (okay, stupid suggestion), reduce the amount of stimulus in your life (T.V, racing around running errands, political talk radio, babysitting your sister's kids, etc.), and generally just suck this pregnancy for all it's worth. Claim exhaustion, kick up your feet, and make everyone else fluff your pillows and fetch your tea.

If all else fails and you're okay with medication, talk to your doctor about pain relief. Tylenol is generally always okay, but if you need something stronger, ask. Headaches are one of those things that tend to get worse as your belly gets bigger, because the hormones get stronger as you progress. Unlike nausea, which (if you're lucky) will usually subside around 12-15 weeks of gestation, headaches may continue to be debilitating without some serious diet or life-style changes, or medication.

The Trouble with Brushing: There's a weird annoyance I want to mention in connection with your first trimester: the possible torment of brushing your teeth. Not an act that one readily associates with pain and suffering, but surging hormones can make this simple daily task a nightmare. For reasons only nature can explain, your body may reject any and all oral stimulation, not just food. Sticking a toothbrush full of paste into your mouth may send you gagging and reeling for the toilet.

I've personally never been afflicted, but an old friend of mine had to brace herself every time she even thought about brushing her teeth. Obviously, you can't go twelve weeks without scrubbing those babies, but how you get through the task is one you will have to experiment with. I think my friend eventually used a little baking soda with water and just quickly ran her finger over her teeth. Gagging was still an ever present occurrence, but at least she managed to keep tooth decay and dragon breath at bay.

You might first try a different paste, maybe an all natural brand with as little added breath freshener as possible. Look for something in an organic or health food store. Open it up, give it a whiff, and if you still gag, you'll know. After that, try just water on a brush, or a little baking soda. If your mouth just won't tolerate a brush, try some gauze or your finger. Worst case scenario, if you think you can tolerate it, you could simply make up a rinse with baking soda and swish it around in your mouth.

Bad Nose, Bad! Yes, your nose knows when you are pregnant and heads straight to misbehaving just as soon as the memo arrives. Hormones cause nosebleeds, clog your sinuses, exaggerate any allergies – you name it. Like everything else in your body, your nasal cavity swells, gets easily irritated, and oh my gosh, does it pick up odors. One of my friends could be tootling around the far end of a two thousand square foot house, yet still be able to sniff out her husband's unthinkable, shocking, and devious exploit and bellow, "Are you cutting a watermelon?!"

What's That Smell?! For the same reason that food aromas put your stomach in a lurch, chemical smells can be ghastly on a pregnant sniffer. I practically faint when my husband breaks out window cleaner. And an old pregger co-worker of mine was vicious when forced to work in a freshly painted office.

Having baby #3 on the way has forced us to sell one of our cars and get a minivan (sigh). My husband keeps asking what I want and my only criteria is that if it's used, it absolutely cannot smell like a cigarette. Always quick to reassure me, he insists that used car dealers put the vehicles through a thorough inspection and cleaning. No worries, honey! We can specify a non-smoking van only.

Well. I don't know whose nicotine nose they use to do the stink test, but the last time I rented a "non-smoking" car from one of these dealers, I may as well have been driving an ashtray. Yes, I was pregnant at the time, and yes, my pregnant nose picks up the stench from a football field away, but the fact of the matter remains. I smelled it and wanted to strangle someone.

No matter the chemical, it's probably best to steer clear of noxious fumes. We are gestating ladies and don't need to be counted among the casualties of our generous lab rat volunteers. Do what you must. Go around quoting, "Prolonged exposure to gasoline fumes has been known to cause cancer in laboratory animals" or whatever you need to avoid exposure and keep your head and belly aches to a minimum.

Nosebleeds – Aaah! Good gravy, these buggers sneak up on you when you least expect it! Right in the middle of an intense meeting, teaching a class, or interviewing babysitters, oh sure, now is a good time. Go for it, Mr. Nose! You go right ahead and gush enough blood to make it look like I lost a bar fight. No problem! My boss is paled and pointing a shaking finger at my face, but hey, no big deal. And by the way, what's with the wimps who can't take a bloody nose?? Good grief! Be a man, for crying out loud.

Always forgetting this nicety of pregnant life until it hits yet again, three times around now, the ol' nose shocks the bejeebies out of me. Here's how it goes: I'm washing my hair in the shower and look down to see red all over my chest, swirling down the drain. Huh. Red. What's red? Shampoo? Soap? Oh crap! That's blood! Where, where is it coming from??! Did my head just explode? Oh wait, I got it. It's my nosebleed welcome committee. Yea! Thanks so much. Don't know if it's the humidity, hot water, or stinky soap, but it looks like you're happy to see me pregnant again! So sweet.

Contrary to when my own bleeds occur, most often the event will coincide with dry, cold weather, which tends to dry out your already compromised nose. Don't panic, because it can look a good deal worse than it really is. Newly pregnant Amy was on the phone with me when I heard a gasp and distant honk as she looked down while driving and realized she was covered in blood. Who knows what kind of swerving was going on at the other end of the phone as she slapped herself silly looking for the cause, shocked and amazed that it was only her nose.

A bit perturbed at my casual, "Oh don't worry about it", she kept repeating, "Are you sure this is normal?? Really?" YES, honey, I am sure this is normal. Break out the Spray-n-Wash or spit on your shirt - then go about your business. Clean it up later. Amy: "I am not spitting on myself! Seriously, spit gets out your own blood???!!" Me: "Well, yeah, I've heard. Give it a whirl – let me know how it goes." Amy: "You are no help!"

Okay, so, back to being helpful. When you get a bleed, just sit up normally (no need to lean back or forward), pinch your nostrils together, and try to stop the flow. If it doesn't stop within 5-10 minutes, or if it looks like you could fill a small bucket with all the blood, call your doctor for recommendations. Otherwise, once it stops, gently clean any excess blood in your nose with a damp cloth - then leave it alone. Don't use any nasal sprays unless your doctor okays a saline or lubricating treatment to cut down the dryness. Other than that, there's nothing to do but wave to the Bloody Nose Welcome Wagon.

Pass Me the Kleenex! Uh. Stuffiness and drainage are a constant in the life of a pregnant woman. Those poor, tender nasal tissues can swell up and stand at full attention for the duration of your hormonal upheaval. Nice, eh? Buy yourself some good tissues with lotion, and don't go ballistic with the blowing. The harder and more often you blow, the more likely you are to irritate or damage your delicate nasal lining. Try to keep your head elevated while you sleep and avoid bending over with your head upside down (buttoning a kid's jacket, putting on shoes, stretching at the gym, drying your hair, etc). When your head is down, blood rushes right in and has a party.

If you happen to get a cold and your nose goes on a flat out strike, try the old fashioned methods of steam and humidifiers first. If that doesn't help relieve some symptoms, call your practitioner for advice on what over-the-counter medication or possibly even vitamin supplements you can take. If you have any medical issues such as high blood pressure, they will need to know this before making any suggestions.

Walking Zombies (Fatigue)

Although briefly mentioned before, this baby bears repeating, as it is probably THE most profound symptom of pregnancy. You're tired after eating breakfast. You're tired after pooping (well, that's a whole different story but we'll get to that later). You're tired if you sneeze twice. You fall asleep while writing an email. You sit down on the couch to watch a little T.V., yet your hand never quite makes it to the remote. Twenty minutes later, your husband walks in asking a confused, "What the heck are you doing?" as he sees you staring blankly at an empty television screen.

I recently lost – yes, lost, just POOF – an entire hour of my morning and had no idea how. I dropped my girls off at preschool, conked on the bed for twenty minutes, and got up to head to the gym. I'm in my car, right on time, doing good, taking care of myself, everything's cool. While patting myself on the back, I happened to glance at the clock. Thirty confused seconds later, dawn broke. I had about ten minutes to get my lazy butt to the school and fetch my kids before the administrator was forced to take them home with her and feed them lunch. What happened to that hour??!!!! That nap felt like five minutes – did I really sleep through my workout time??

The fatigue and weariness associated with gestation is very nearly frightening – well, for the five minutes a day that you're awake and alert, anyway. You vacillate between feeling guilty for being so useless, and being so tired that you could care less what others think. (My vote will always fall in the second category.) Making the placenta and getting that little critter formed is no small potatoes. You may not be covered in sweat, scratches, or bruises, and you may not have much to show for your three months of intensive labor, but believe me, your body is working at maximum potential. Anyone who doesn't understand or sympathize can just stuff it.

There's no real cure for getting over the fatigue. You can stay in bed all day long yet still have to drag your weary butt into the bathroom and shower. Arms and legs will still feel full of lead, and lungs will still protest anything more than a walk to the fridge. Just get used to the fact that you are going to answer your phone completely out of breath only to inform the concerned caller that you were simply cutting apples or folding laundry.

Your best bet is to stay on your normal routine – just modify it to squeeze in naps or rest. Collapse on the couch when you get home from work, go to bed an hour or two early, and sleep in when you can. With the exception of exercise (which is almost always a good thing), cut out any and all unnecessary tootles around town. And forget dashing to a friend's house for the latest gossip unless you can crash on her couch while she gabs away in your half-asleep ear.

A Tiny Bit of Caffeine, Please? Many women, especially by the second or third pregnancy, ease up on the caffeine ban in order to get an energy boost. During my first pregnancy, if you'd argued that one cup of coffee per day is acceptable, I would have choked on my skinless, organic, hormone-free chicken. But this number three has knocked me so silly that I actually succumb to a short cola (and eat nice, deep-*fried* chicken) once every two or three weeks. One of my friends allows her third-time-pregnant-self a guilt-free cola every day, and shockingly, she claims everything is ticking along just fine.

Now, I'm certainly not recommending that you follow in our footsteps. Caffeine is a stimulant, bad for your baby, bad for your pregnancy, and bad for your health. I'm only saying that if you are desperate for a pick-me-up, don't load yourself with guilt along with the sugar and other no-no's that go into caffeinated drinks. Just keep it to a minimum and vow to do better tomorrow.

Oouch! (Pain Down Low)

There are generally two causes of the strange and sometimes alarming pelvic or lower abdominal pain. As far as cramping pain goes, it's most likely due to the stretching uterus and ligaments. The pain can be on one or both sides and usually feels like a low sharp jab when you make sudden movements or first get out of bed. Unless you're bleeding or the pain is quite unbearable, don't be too anxious about it. As with all things, if you need reassurance, call your caregiver. It's better to be safe than sorry.

Even this third time around, I constantly worried about a miscarriage or tubal pregnancy (an embryo that implants in one of the fallopian tubes). For both concerns, I was consistently put off by my doc. If there is no bleeding or great pain, I would just have to wait until my eight-week sonogram. Doctors can't do much to ease your mind until they can really see what's going on – and that's right around eight weeks. Many doctors will do a "dating sono" around this time to get an accurate due date, check for a nice strong heartbeat, and confirm how many critters you've got cooking. Until then, try to relax and let Mother Nature do her thing.

The other rather perplexing discomfort in your pelvic region is also due to muscles changes. Your hips or tailbone may ache, and in this case, it's due to relaxing muscles and ligaments. Your body does all sorts of spreading and contorting in preparation for birth, and there's not much to do about it. Your body will do what it needs to do no matter how much you protest to the contrary.

Sometimes in late pregnancy you'll feel a searing, knife-jabbing, hot-poker kind of pain right where it counts (which happens to be your cervix). This pain is a catch-your-breath-stop-and-yell kind of torture. If you aren't actually in labor, which can be a similar experience, this nuisance pain can be due to stretching *nerves* (yeah, love that). If you've never had a nerve stretch, pray you never do. The baby's head pounds your cervix and those poor little nerves have nowhere to go – YOUCH!

Many of these pains aren't anything you can *do* much about, except sit down or slow down. Aching bones and stretching "things" are just part of the process your body must go through. Rest always seems to be the best remedy for me. My second kid was sunny side up at birth and knocked my tailbone for a loop. A posterior position of the baby (face up) during delivery puts more pressure on your tailbone. In my case, it took about a full year to feel normal again. Now that I'm pregnant again, the old girl is declaring her dissent. The pressure of my growing uterus makes even walking unbearable sometimes - and the only solution is rest. So let's kick back, ladies! Grab a book and some ice cream, and live it up!

Twenty Four Pounds of Boob Comin' Through!

Scaring you is not high on my to-do list, but I'm here to dish out the honest truth, so hold your breath and prepare. Here's a few good descriptors: huge, mongo, outrageous, nipples the size of compact discs, blue alien veins, and let's see…did I say huge? As in, they have GOT to be 12 pounds each. Those babies are freaking unreal.

On the bright side, all this Amazon-booby business could mean a great deal of fun if hubby is into that sort of thing. My friend's husband thought it rather cool when her gargantuan breasts starting gushing colostrum during sex. (Yes, that actually happens.) Personally, I give it the ol' pause and "huh" as weirdness overwhelms excitement, but hey, whatever. Unfortunately, if you don't happen to enjoy this voluptuous part of your pregnancy, it only leaves you staring at your naked body in confusion and fright.

Gimmie a Big One! The first order of business is a bra. And sorry honey, but you're going to have to give up sexy for comfort. Unless, of course, you think sticking balloons in a size 38 double G zebra print is sexy. We are moms-to-be and need to get over ourselves and our need to be cute. There is no "cute" in pregnant boobs. (Unless you were flat-chested to begin with – in which case, enjoy the goods.)

So buy a couple of good bras. I know you will hate me forever and ever, but go to an actual maternity store and fit yourself with a nice stretchy job that will grow and adjust with you. You will get over the ugliness, I promise! Try first for an increase in cup size, not jump in ribcage measurement. For instance, if you normally wear a 34B, try a 34C, then a 34D and DD before you move up to a size 36. The hope is that your boobs are the only thing that will get bigger, not your entire torso. Your ribcage generally does expand, however, so you may end up a number size (or two or three, who's counting?) bigger before all is said and done. Don't worry about this or attribute it to fat. Attribute it to Mother Nature's expansion project.

Down Baby, Down! Now, the only other thing you need to worry about in the bra department (you're gonna love this) is having nipples that refuse to "stand down." Sometimes those little guys just can't seem to get out of an erect mode, showing through 90% of the bras you try on. This creates a - how shall we say it - "non-motherly" look. If you're catching my drift and sharing my pain, get a bra with lots of nice padding. Just what you need to bust right out of your shirts.

While disconcerting at first, your belly will eventually get so big that those monstrous boobs will pale in comparison. Until then, protect and support those babies with all you've got. Yes, they'll be I'm-going-to-die sore, and if someone so much as brushes up against your delicate darlings, you'll roar in agony and start throwing punches. The good news is, like nausea, this unbearable pain should diminish and pass with initiation into the second trimester. Your mammoth knockers will still be a nuisance to manage and may get hot enough to fry eggs, but they shouldn't be horribly tender.

Growing Extra Boobs: You think I joke, but this is absolutely the most taboo thing I've ever heard – and totally true. Some people (men included) are born with supernumerary nipples. They appear as skin tags, tiny moles, or just some general don't-really-know-what-that-thing-is harmless lesion. For pregnant women, the hormone surge will sometimes cause them to 'pop out,' making you gasp, "Damn, what IS that?!" In rare cases, two will develop and actually function as milk duds. Most of the time they appear somewhere under your regular nipple on your torso, but other places seem to be just as jolly for the little guys as well. Sometimes you will grow an extra nipple when pregnant, but it won't mature into a full-fledged, functioning breast. Apparently it's somewhat common, with some people growing two extra nipples/breasts on each side. Who knew!

I only know of two women with this condition. Luckily (for us, anyway) one of them had an extreme case to share. So if you fall anywhere along the spectrum, big hugs. You are not alone!! We are here, honey; your personal support group. Here's Rachel's story: So, she's a few months pregnant when she noticed a small brown line under her armpit. After several weeks the line morphed into a little bump. Then she got a matching brown line under her other armpit, which turned into a twin bump. She figured they were weird pregnancy skintabs or something, no big deal. Well, several weeks later a nice, rosy pink circle appeared around each bump, making it look eerily familiar. Yikes. So she showed them to her OB-GYN, who happily proclaimed, "Congratulations! You're a mammal!"

Okay. Let us take a moment, shall we? Please raise your hand if you think this helped. Because I'm clueless. Happy, chipper people make me cringe to begin with. So having a medical authority cheerily tell you congrats, when you could just as well be growing a couple of horns, is beyond stupid. Can we give a collective snort here, ladies? This dude just told our girlfriend that she's a warm-blooded vertebrate animal of the class Mammalia among the ranks of whales, carnivores, rodents, bats, and primates. Gee. Thanks.

So back to the story. Lo and behold, it was two "auxiliary breasts" sprouting up to make sure old babe-ums got enough milk. Pretty shocking and not super cute, but at least they were small. That is, until the baby was born and milk started coming in. Then the two invaders filled up with milk just like regular ol' boobies. They could even make a good squirt across a room. Luckily they shrunk immensely after Rachel stopped breastfeeding but didn't go away completely. Now, where you go with this information, I'm sure I don't know, but you can't say I didn't warn you.

One Hairy Monster

A little less frightening topic (sort of), pregnancy hair can be a source of great joy. Many women (count me out) report having thick and luxurious locks during the forty weeks of gestation (who are you people, anyway??) They then complain when it falls out in clumps after giving birth, but take it while you can. Affecting every square inch of your body, those hormones can do wonders for a limp do.

The only down side to having hormones that go bananas on your head is that they go ape everywhere else too – and I mean you'll look like an ape. Hair sprouts from nipples (charming) that are already such a foreign color and size that you'll stay awake at night wondering if you're normal. Leg hair gets bushy and murders your razors. Pubic hair gets so out of control that nothing short of a lawn mower will do the trick. And you might even find yourself sprouting obnoxious looking whiskers all over your belly, face, and rectum. LOVE it!!! Just yesterday, I spied and nixed a two-inch long strand poking out of the top of my foot. How it got there, I'll never know, but the rest of the day was drowned in depression. A TWO inch hair??!! On my FOOT? Just...how???!!

Pregnancies number one and two had me taking desperate measures as I raced to the drug store to buy the first heavy-duty hair removal kit I could find. Twenty minutes later I'm lathering up my belly with green goo, sticking a square patch of cotton cloth over it, and ripping off all unsightly fuzz with crazed fervor. Did it work? Yes. Did I scream in anguish? Yes. And as a result of those experiments, this time around I'm sticking to razors and tweezers.

Poop & Grapes (Bowels and Hemorrhoids)

There are many women who claim to have no bowel trouble whatsoever during pregnancy (I don't know you, but I hate your lying ass - literally). But those of us who aren't so lucky (or lack any sense of dignity) will yammer our woes to anyone who will listen. I mean, sheesh! We must spend half of the day in the bathroom! You really feel the need to go, but get stuck on the toilet with body parts refusing to cooperate. This leads to overkill pushing and the dreaded "H" word.

Hemorrhoids are terrifying and disgusting. Take my advice and do all you can to avoid the torture. Otherwise, you'll be forced to break out the Preparation H, and it will be a very sad day indeed. Get into the habit of eating tons of fiber to head off any trouble. Dietary fiber alone may not be enough, but at least you can start the ball rolling.

Eat loads of fresh fruit, raw vegetables, leafy greens, and bran. Munch on apples, prunes, grapes, oranges with tons of white skin still on them, kidney beans, lentils, sweet potatoes, broccoli, or anything with a nice fiberous skin. Drink prune and apple juice (you can mix the two to make it taste better) and plenty of water or Gatorade.

Now, how do you know if you actually have a nasty butt grape? Several clues will key you in. Your bowel movements could be accompanied by a lovely spurt of blood. Or the pain of the event might cause an anguished howl to echo throughout your office building. You could have some general (or horrible) itchiness, burning, or discomfort on the ol' keister. If you're in the shower and happen to feel some swelling or puffy lumps, that's another good indicator. And, if you are brave enough to look (I wouldn't advise – it takes several mirrors and bending in ways you shouldn't bend), you will see some rather frightening looking bulges, inflammation, or pea-to-marble size clumps of swollen flesh on your rectum. Jumping Jehosaphat, just kill me!!

All this may sound scary enough to start pleading with God, but really, more people suffer from it (and survive) than you'll ever know. It's just not a subject one talks about. There's something about bowels and rectum trouble that makes people shy away from the topic. Imagine that! Until you're old enough that your innards conk out and things just don't work the way they should, your peers and friends will keep tight-lipped about their anal troubles and bowel movements. And frankly, it seems to me that life is better that way.

So, once you've made a fair assumption that hemorrhoids are the trouble (or you're brave enough to have your doctor check), the next step is easing the discomfort and getting those bowels going. Getting more fiber should help move things along, but you could still end up with a horrid case of cement butt and need more aggressive forms of relief. And for me, turning to those basic pregnancy guides for advice left me screeching in frustration. Nonstop I-need-to-barf didn't motivate me to stuff my face with more nasty food for relief.

Check with your doctor or midwife for different options, but my personal favorite was Metamucil tablets. The only thing I had to choke down with the pills was a glass of water, and that was much better than the alternative. You do have to take a seemingly large amount of tablets per day, but it works. Your practitioner may also recommend Milk of Magnesia, which is generally safe, or they may even go so far as to allow you to have Colace.

Do some research online and ask your doctor about straight magnesium supplements. Aside from being a great poop-inducer, recent research indicates it's a natural relaxer – possibly reducing the incidence of preeclampsia, poor fetal growth, premature labor contractions, leg cramps, insomnia, stress, and irregular heartbeat. It may also help regulate blood sugar and cholesterol levels. (Shit, with all this new information, please ask me how happy I am to have learned it AFTER passing all those dadgum, gi-normous rocks in my colon!) Whatever method you choose, you may have to experiment a bit to get the dosage right, and the entire ordeal may end up quite ugly, but it's just another little unpleasantry in the life of a pregger.

As for immediate relief of hemorrhoid discomforts, first try a sitz bath. Or lie on your side and prop up your hips to relieve some of the pressure on your rear. The only problem with boosting the hips is that if you happen to also need head elevation due to heartburn, you'll end up a human pretzel. Not a good thing.

Your other options are prescription or over the counter creams like Preparation H or Anusol, but make sure and check with the big D on this one. The sheer mortification of needing a hemorrhoid cream is cry-worthy, I know. But I can almost promise that the pregnant lady next door has them too. It's a total actress job if she's glowing and happy and acts like her bum-button isn't killing her.

So okay! Time to wrap up life in the first trimester! It can give you quite a few hiccups, or none at all. If you're sailing through without a hitch, be thankful and don't worry. It doesn't mean anything is wrong (it just means the rest of us HATE you). Every person is different, and every pregnancy is different. When you're miserable and sick you think, "Why, *why* me?!" Yet when you feel great you frantically wonder, "Is everything okay?" There's no getting around the constant doubt, anxiety, and fear, no matter how good or bad you feel. Either way, just remember that with each passing day, you're getting closer to holding a precious little angel in your arms. Concentrate on that and let your body do the rest!

Chapter Three: One Flew Over the Cuckoo's Nest

When you're pregnant, you tend to go a little psycho. In fact, for many women, this crazed state of mind is what first clues them in that a tiny someone may be showing up for dinner in the next nine months. That is, in fact, exactly how I came to suspect my own little condition.

Rooting around inside a giant tube slide, I was trying to locate my screaming child at the park. Along comes another (supervisor-less) little chick-a-dee, barking at me to watch him climb the monkey bars. "Hey lady, wanna watch me? Look at me! Lady, wanna see what I can do? Watch me, watch me!"

After winding my way through ten feet of toddler-sized tube, I finally managed to locate my child and drag her far enough to poke my head out of the entrapment. Following me like a duckling, here's this same little kid, two inches from my nose, continuing to pester me for attention. Snap-a-roo time! Get out of my face and SHUT UP! Five seconds after barking, "Noooo! I can't watch you right now!" I thought, "Uh-oh." I was only about two days late for my period, but it's one of those things where you just *know*.

Honey, once you've been there and done that enough, you understand that pregnancy hormones make you do strange things. Sure, other people's kids may not get the endless adoration your own do, but for Pete's sake! As a mother, you tend to welcome all lost sheep into your own flock (as long as they aren't biting, back-talking, or kicking little heathens). This time, however, the lost lamb got a snarl. And that's just plain weird.

When gestating, every ounce of your being is focused on your belly whether you actually realize it or not. *You* may not know you're pregnant, but your body does. This means you'll start acting crazy. Pronto. Then, once you've confirmed your body is indeed morphing with child, your brain shuts all unnecessary doors, consuming your attention for the next nine months. Yesterday you were obsessed with getting that proposal written for the big board meeting. Today, all you care about is heading straight to the nearest mall to look for layettes and maternity clothes – all the while growling at anyone who dares defy your mood.

Sorry my dear, this crazy-B (as in Bleep!) business happens to the best of us. Kid you not, I once had a pregnant woman holler "dummy!" when I gave her the right of way. No joke, I'm in my car, see her walking and about to cross the street, so I stop and wave her across. We go back and forth a couple of times with "no, you go" "no, no, you go first" – and she finally stomps across the street in disgust and growls, "dummy!" ??!!!

What the *&^%??! My window was down, there was no one else around, so the bark was clearly for me, but - why?? It was a stop sign! Pregnant pedestrians clearly have the right of way! I really have no freaking clue - just went home and cried. To my husband, on the other hand, it was clear as day. "She was pregnant? Well, there's your answer." HUH?? Seriously ladies, you can't go around calling people "dummy" for being nice or screaming at store clerks for bagging your groceries wrong. _I_ don't do that. Oh crap. I _don't_ do that, do I??

Baby Don't Care

When the euphoria wears off, the first big anxiety takes over all thoughts: the initial slap in the face that some mighty big changes are going to happen. The life you've spent years creating and getting comfortable with must now accommodate another tiny, yet very intolerant, human being. You may initially think this little creature will mold very nicely into your life, quickly learning to respect you and your mate's sleep, work schedule, play schedule, and the dog's ownership of the couch. All will be hunky-dory.

At some point, however, reality will seep in as you realize that this little creature will not give a rat's ass how much sleep you need, how important that work deadline is, or, for that matter, the fact that you need to shower, eat, or pee. No, this little slave-driver in the making will not care. He will, in fact, have you running around the house like a chicken with your head cut off trying to keep up with feeding, diapering, gas, baths, spit-up, and all the other I-have-no-earthly-idea-what-the-heck-this-kid-is-crying-about needs. You will soon find that not only will this kid *not* mold into what you consider a workable routine, he will determine what chores do (and don't) get done around your house, how much you do (and don't) eat, and how much sex you are (and aren't) having.

Light bulbs start clicking a bit sooner if you had a difficult first trimester and came to terms with how much havoc a tiny little fetus can wreak on your body and life. The critter isn't even out and howling yet, and you've had to rearrange you life just to make it through the day without passing out. So at some point you begin to realize how different your life will be and how scary that reality is. Thus begins your I-can't-concentrate-on-anything-else mental and emotional changes.

Impulse Rules!

Loss of Control and Anxiety: Even if you are nothing but thrilled with your impending arrival, hormones alone will put you in a lurch. Expect all sorts of out-of-character weeping, yelling, snapping, and fretting. Add in all the other normal worries regarding furniture, hospitals, doctors, birthing plans, dreams of bonding and baby accessories, and you've got a recipe for Mommy Madness. There is just no more room in your crowded brain for logic or formerly important issues. You are having a baby. What in the Universe could possibly be more important than that?

Food - Now! One of the main reasons for loss of control in the life of the gestating lady is hunger. I really don't know what it is, but you can be walking along, having a nice conversation with your mate when all of a sudden, IT hits you like a brick: the overwhelming urge to eat before you kill someone. It's so intense that you're a sobbing puddle of mush if you don't get some sustenance within two minutes. Any normal person would calmly think, "Ah. Guess I'm getting a little hungry. I'll see about eating just as soon as I finish up this email." Well, listen up all ye women with child! You can't do that. Don't put it off as you normally would because this is not something you can ignore and get over. Make an immediate change of itinerary and start waddling yourself to the nearest refrigerator, salad bar, or cafeteria. Do it quick before someone gets hurt.

Get yourself a quick degree in pregnancy-smarts: plan ahead and keep snacks on you at all times. You'll have to get used to this anyway, as little kids are eating and pooping machines and consume about as much as a full-grown hobbit. Once you start toting around baby chicks, get ready. They have their mouth open every time they aren't sprinting or high-speed crawling away from you.

I guess that's where this compulsion to eat comes from. The same child that will soon be demanding every Cheerio and granola bar you can stuff into his mouth is just exerting his power a little early. And being the great Mommies that we are, we will, of course, obey every eating command. Everyone knows that a Mommy's first concern is making sure that no offspring of *hers* goes hungry!

Peeing: Another area of physical need that will have you knocking over old ladies on the way to your destination is the extreme need to pee. With your average, non-pregnant person, the need to relieve your bladder is a gradual onset of intensity. For a pregnant woman, however, there are two states of bladder awareness: *empty* and *about-to-burst.* It's as if the baby in your belly is in control of the pee switch, and he's not paying attention half the time. Only after your bladder is bulging and infringing on his twirling space, does he flip the switch and send the message to your brain that you have got to go – NOW.

There will also be times when the little darling will not tolerate even one ounce of urine pressing against your uterus, forcing his toes to squish up his nose. So he'll flip the switch every ten minutes just to make sure his nasal cavity doesn't come out looking like a chimpanzee's. While this a good thing, all in all, it still keeps the gestating vessel hopping from one toilet to the next shouting, "Sweet mother of Abraham Lincoln, *get out of my way!*" Boy, if that doesn't make for a ferocious fight, should anyone claim a more urgent need and deny a pregnant woman her place on the porcelain.

"I Don't Know Why!" If an immediate physical need or depression over your morphing body doesn't get your guitar strumming, just plain old hormones will send you running for the tissue with no clue as to why. As big a deal as being *physically* pregnant is, mentally you feel like a gigantic science experiment, happy as a chipmunk one minute and glaring and snarling the next.

The most confusing part of it all is that you have no ability to reason your way through the madness. You may find yourself raging over an inability to get your sock on fast enough, or sobbing when you realize you're almost out of your favorite nail polish. What the hell?! Throw hubby in there getting upset with you for letting the car run out of gas, and shit - we're just a pile of heaping, bawling mush.

The "I don't know why" aspect of pregnancy breakdowns is hard enough as it is, but even more challenging is trying to convince your husband that this is a normal. Men, being the giant testosterone-making creatures they are, will never, ever, in two million years, understand the emotional roller coaster you're on. It's taken male doctors eons to even believe that nausea is an actual physical symptom of pregnancy. (Where's my hot poker?! Anyone got a cattle prod?) How long do you think it will take them to understand the dynamics of why we act so crazy when our baby's cooking?

I still can't convince my husband that a drop in blood sugar renders a person out of control, because he's never experienced it. Granted, he is very tolerant of my ranting and raving while pregnant, so hey, this is no hubby-bashing gig. I'm only saying that when the event is confusing enough that *we* can't explain it, good luck getting hubby to empathize. Just beg him in your good moments to be patient and kind and run out to get you chocolate cake or whatever your heart desires whenever you start to whimper. Tell him not to ask or argue because you will never be able to provide him with a satisfactory answer. And if you are so inclined, inform him that this Michelle Smith lady promises you will be your rational self again once the kid is out and the hormones aren't flooding you onto Noah's Ark.

Mirror, Mirror You Lying Dog!

Not only has Mother Nature conned you into thinking this pregnancy thing was nothing but a trip to bliss-land, but she's transformed your former self into a stranger. Gone are the days of carefree trips to the coffee shop, shopping for sexy lingerie, or even having a hormonally-balanced day. You wake up each morning and cringe as you look in the mirror and see dimples and fat forming where it never dared before. Not to mention boobs that resemble a veiny blue roadmap (with a huge bulls eye) and a belly that, while kind of cute in the beginning, is starting to look freakish.

Now, all you women who maintain your petite and lovely frames while pregnant, bear with me, as the rest of us are not blessed with your genetics. I actually did maintain a rather small and dimple-free body with my first pregnancy. Frolicking at the beach five weeks before delivery, people would gush, "Gosh, I didn't even realize you were pregnant until you turned to the side!" (Thank you, Mr. Very-expensive-black-bathing-suit.) A tiny 23 pounds bigger (aah, the glory days) and tanned like a golden Thanksgiving turkey, I even managed to tick my sister off by dazzling everyone in the delivery room with my glowing skin, bright smile, and dark-circle-free eyes.

But wait! Life and age soon wrecked it all, so don't assume the gloat switch has flipped. Oh contraire, this sickening story is only shared as a reality check. You may be confident that it's all in how you take care of yourself or that you are destined to be among the great gestators of our time. If it happens that way, I'm all too happy for you, but it might be wise to keep Captain Cocky on a shelf.

Yeah, sure, you could very well end up a clone of Mrs. Fancy Pants at my gym. She's a tall, disgustingly gorgeous brunette working on baby #4. At eight months, you can still barely notice the tiny lump in her abdomen. She continues to strut around in bike shorts, showing off legs that could knock out the best of us with one swift kick. She happens to do this pregnancy thing well, and my only comment (behind clenched teeth) is, "more power to you." I'm only saying that most of us can't take the continual body-whipping that baby making demands. If you happen to get a little too self-assured, you may be in for a big thwack when baby #2 hits.

This brings us to my point about the surprises of body changes, especially with multiple pregnancies. By the time my second child was on the way, my husband and I had this fantastic family. We had no idea that a second run around the block would be any different. Initially sure of ourselves, we were blind-sided by the fact that I didn't breeze through the next nine months with little more trouble than having to buy a couple more pairs of maternity pants. The well-deserved butt-kicking came in the form of bulging varicose veins and back muscles so messed up that I was bed-ridden for several weeks. By the time baby #2 popped out, I was a waddling, limping, crippled fool.

Given all this body maiming, depression was a given by the time I was six or seven months into the whole ordeal. It's just plain bewildering when your body acts so bizarre. In retrospect, it's not so horrible a transformation. But when you're going through it, you must allow yourself the freedom to embrace your new self and not get so overwhelmed with the sudden weight gain and swollen belly.

Remember, you are MAKING an entirely new human being. Cut yourself a little slack. It may take a while, but I promise, if you are determined, you *will* shrink back to your former self. In the meantime, feel free to throw the occasional pity party. In fact, get together with other pregnant women and share your misery. Life is great when you find that your troubles really aren't that bad compared to theirs. Horrible as it is, we often feel better when we compare ourselves to others and realize that we are not alone in our despair, or that things could be a heck of a lot worse.

Freddy Krueger's a Kitten (Fears)

Amazing that such a tiny creature can start an avalanche of fright and worry. As soon as you find out you're going to be someone's mother, a wave of "what if's" keep your mind going for hours each day. From "what if my husband won't love me" to "what if I get too fat," we'll cover some of the most frequent fears that moms-to-be go through every single day.

Fear of Miscarriage: I touched on this a bit earlier with my own fears of a tubal pregnancy, but it bears elaboration. From the moment you discover that cells are dividing and forming, you will have an automatic attachment to your future baby. Sheer instinct and force of nature makes us insanely protective and emotionally dedicated to our upcoming arrival. We don't even know this little person, but will do our utmost to make sure he makes a grand appearance on this planet, alive and well.

Miscarriage is a very real fear, but a statistically low probability. I have certainly had my share of friends who have miscarried – young *and* over 35 (by the way, I don't consider that "old" by any stretch of the imagination). But the threat of losing your baby is something you can't do much about.

If you have a high-risk pregnancy, just follow doctor's orders and do your best to ensure a positive outcome. You can get plenty of rest, avoid exercise, take any necessary medications – the whole ball of wax. What I've found, however, is that for the most part, nature is in charge here. Medical technology can certainly help us along in our quest to achieve conception. To some degree, it can even get us through a pregnancy that by all accounts shouldn't have made it. But there are many aspects of gestating that doctors just can't fix or change.

For whatever reason, your body is the big decision maker here. In most cases, you will have absolutely no control over whether or not your body rejects the embryo. There are women who get pregnant without knowing it, and put themselves through the ringer with diet, exercise, stress, caffeine, drugs, and a host of other horrible things. Yet nine months later, out pops this gorgeous baby, much to the amazement of everyone involved. Then there are those who do nothing but tiptoe around the house, and they still miscarry. It's one big mystery.

I happen to think that your body will give you clues if you're in danger of miscarriage, and there isn't a smidgen of anything you can do about it except kick your activity level down a notch and hit the bed. I know many people will spot early in pregnancy. I did with my first kid. And to me, that's your body's way of saying, "Okay, need you to slow down here!" The first thing a doctor will tell you is to go to bed, put your feet up, and rest.

Now, when it comes to having a perfectly healthy pregnancy and doing your best to ensure the baby's the safety, there are limits to what you can realistically do. You can certainly slow down a hair if you've been too active, but when lacking real risk factors for miscarriage, there is no need to stop your life, stay in bed, and simply *will* this child to survive. Chances are incredibly good that he will, despite you and your anxiety.

My advice is to let go, be at peace with Mother Nature, and let her do the walking and talking. Try to enjoy your new status. There are so many wonderful aspects of pregnancy (although you wouldn't know it with all the griping I've been doing) that there is absolutely no need for you to worry yourself into a frenzy over something that probably won't happen. It's much better to focus on the positive and do what you can to take excellent care of yourself. That is something you *do* have control over.

Fear of Becoming a Whale: Ah yes, the eternal question; "What if I gain too much weight?" This is probably the biggest obsession with pregnant women. Whether we admit it or not, we're constantly scrutinizing other pregnant women, eavesdropping, and doing all we can to make ourselves feel better about scarfing down every hamburger, chip, and sweet morsel we can find.

I am now safely to the point in my own pregnancy where any and all food is appealing. Just a couple of nights ago (*after* dinner, mind you) I made an obnoxious plate of hotdogs doused with cheese and mustard. It didn't even occur to me how fattening the whole thing was until my husband gave me the raised eyebrow. I immediately felt guilty – but not so guilty that I didn't gobble down every last bite of dog. And shame be damned, I washed it all down with cherry vanilla ice cream, because I NEED SOME CALCIUM, please.

Fear of getting fat is a persistent, looming evil that stalks us all with great delight. It doesn't matter how healthy you were before, or what the scales stopped at before you got knocked up. Each and every time you go to the doctor's office and step on that loathsome number genie, you're ridden with panic and doubt.

Most every pregnancy book you open says 25-35 pounds of weight gain is acceptable: 25 being for women who were a bit heavy before they got pregnant, and closer to 35 pounds for those skinny little toothpicks who make us scrunch up our noses and wonder how we can voodoo some cottage cheese onto their rottenly beautiful legs.

Now, depending on your doctor, you may or may not get weight lectures. My friend Amy had a drill sergeant for an OB, and this unkindly woman insisted that my tall and lean friend stick to 5 pounds of weight gain for the first *20 weeks*. Amy was, of course, in a panic when she gained 7 measly pounds, terrified that she was headed straight for the beach to join the whales. Upon hearing this ridiculous dilemma, my first question was, "Has this meathead doctor of yours ever been pregnant?" The answer? Of course not. What research this woman pulled her numbers from, I will never know, but from then on out I blasted this doctor every chance I got (and Amy did change to a different one, thank heavens). A *woman* too! Sheesh. Where's the sympathy? Where's the love?

You all know the general guidelines for weight gain, so you won't hear it again here. But no matter how much you put on, there are two things I have found to be true. First, a gradual increase in weight, as opposed to jumps and spurts, gives us time to adjust to the change without feeling so horribly out of sync. Second, with the exception of completely out of control eating, most women will pretty much gain the same amount of weight for each pregnancy, and your body will pretty much do what it wants to do, regardless of your input or objection. There are those women who consistently put on 40-50 pounds and there are those who consistently stick to the puny 25.

Even outside of pregnancy, weight is such a constant struggle with many women that it's almost useless to fight it while you're pregnant. This is not to say that you should bury your face in the fridge and only come out for air, but do your best and leave it at that. Pregnancy is not the time to diet and it's not the time to wallow in self-pity because you're gaining 30 pounds – you're supposed to. Sure, it's dang uncomfortable, and there's the lingering fear of being unable to take it off once the baby arrives, but you can cross that bridge when you come to it. For now, just do your best to keep processed foods, sugar, and fat intake to a minimum, and go on with life, proud, plump, and happy.

Honey, Do I Look Fat? Fear that your husband won't find you attractive is, well, not so unjustified. Here you are, looking like you swallowed a melon (or a basketball), your feet and face swell beyond recognition, and your emotional state leaves hubby walking on eggshells. However, what will surprise many of you is that for the first eight months of this gig, your husband may actually be all over you with desire. To him, the voluptuous boobs and curvy new body can be like getting a whole new sex partner with no fear of wrath from his wife. What's even better is that sex can be a brand new source of fun and excitement for you *both* (more on that later).

Once you hit the last month of your journey, you need not worry what hubby thinks. Either the sheer logistics of sex will baffle you both into giving up, or you'll be so miserable that you won't give a flip what he thinks. As long as he shows up for the birth and takes your hand squeezing, cussing, and pushing like a champ, you'll quickly forget that he's the miserable sod who got you into this mess. Soon enough, you'll both be gazing at your fabulous creation and making so many goo-goo faces that neither one of you will even remember your former pheromone woes.

How Bad Will Labor Hurt?! The fear of labor won't hit you hard until you're nearing the end, but it will still be a nagging dread throughout your entire pregnancy. I've said it before and I'll say it again – you can read every pregnancy book on the planet and do your best to prepare for your big day, but you absolutely will not know how labor will affect you until you're there. Be my guest in reading all those books because it will familiarize you with many of the common experiences, but don't expect or assume too much.

Now, for the big question: "How much does it hurt?" Again, I reiterate myself – you won't know until you're there. For the most part, the answer is emphatically "like a bitch," but as for where and how much, that's up to Mother Nature. We'll get more detailed on specifics later, but for now, trust me when I tell you that the fear and anticipation is worse than the event itself. Labor is definitely a wild ride, but I promise, you will forget the pain. Once it's over, you may say, "Whew, that sucked!" but you will finally understand that fear and dread do nothing and need not be any part of the labor equation. You will make it through and you will even want another kid somewhere down the road. Yes siree, bub. It will happen.

Ten Fingers and Toes: Fear of something being wrong with the baby is probably the biggest fear most pregnant women have. Our dreams of having a beautiful, healthy baby are constantly marred by "what if..." When you have certain risk factors for having a baby with genetic or physical challenges, believe me, your doctor will work with you to get all the appropriate testing and counseling you need. I know you won't listen, but I'll tell you again that your chances of actually having a baby with problems are so low that it's really not worth worrying about. If it happens, it happens. You might as well quit fretting about it and deal *if* it ever comes up. Otherwise, you are wasting precious day-dreaming space in your brain worrying about something that probably won't be an issue.

Now, if you are having a perfectly normal and healthy pregnancy, and you have no risk factors for any problems, please do us all a favor and chill! Going through fears regarding the health and safety of your baby is so normal that it only convinces me of your fantastic Mommy potential. Listen girlfriend, little Baby is happy as a clam, floating around your innards and kicking the tar out of your bladder. Give it a rest and breathe!

What if I Suck at Parenting? Practically every woman alive has some issue with one or both parents. Future parents idealize perfect childrearing and don't want to make the same mistakes as their own parents. Even if you feel nothing but sheer joy and love flowing between you and your parents, there is bound to be some anxiety over whether or not you will be able to raise your own child as well, or whether you can possibly provide all the love, attention, time, and care a newborn needs.

I happen to think this particular fear is a good one; it puts us on high alert. We've all seen or heard horror stories regarding the care of children, and it confounds us how people are so callous with the well being of such an innocent creature in their hands. If you had *no* fears about being a great parent, I might actually be concerned. Granted, some people are so naturally cheery and relaxed that this whole parenting thing is something to enjoy and be taken in stride. But for the rest of us, worry is a reality check. If you're like me and worry yourself into therapy over doing the right thing, it tells me that (a) you get the seriousness of your duty as a parent and (b) you will probably be awesome at it.

Suffice it to say that for now, all you need to do is be grateful for your instincts, trust your ability and common sense, and let everything come what may. I hate to break the news to you, but you will not be a perfect parent – nobody is. But that's the beauty of it. Children need to know, and will learn from you, that they, too, are not perfect but can grow up to be wonderful, loving, thoughtful, productive, and happy – just like you!

A Litter of Pups: We all go through a phase of getting so big that we're convinced there must be a litter of pups in there. But the fears are about 97% unfounded. Gestational bloating (especially with subsequent pregnancies) is often so horrid that you're throwing on maternity clothes before you've even told people you're pregnant. (Mercy.) Once you get a sonogram at about eight weeks or so, all fears can either be put aside or thrown into the fire. Worry about it then.

Every once in a great while, you'll get a bomb thrown your way, but usually only if you've run the gamut of fertilization treatments. I once met a guy who said his wife went in for her eight-week sono and was told that two babies were on the way. Halfway through her pregnancy, she got another little surprise as baby #3 decided to introduce himself when the cameras were rolling. Talk about shock! Two is doable, but three out-numbers you. Crimony! You may as well have four or five buns cooking. I'd throw in the towel and call my therapist.

If you do happen to get the glorious news that more than one baby is on the way, don't freak out just yet. While I haven't met many women who are actually pregnant with multiple babies, I do know several who already have them – and you know what? Everything turned out just fine. If this is your first pregnancy, so much the better because once those babies arrive, you won't have any prior knowledge of how things are supposed to be, and you won't have any other kids to worry about. You will learn as you go, plug along, and do just great. If it's a subsequent pregnancy, you'll at least have some idea of what to expect and can prepare yourself for double-duty.

La-La Land

I Don't Remember That! One of the great mysteries of being pregnant and having children is the memory loss that accompanies the event. Perhaps you are so distracted that you can't listen to what people tell you in the first place, or perhaps all firing neurons are aiming toward your belly. Whatever the reason, we Mommies tend to get a little on the absent-minded side. Laugh all you want, but believe me, you'll get yours. One day you'll be in court trying the case of your life and won't be able to recall the specifics of a bullet entry (have I been watching too much T.V.?) Instead, all you can concentrate on is trying to stifle a burp or squeeze your butt cheeks together to keep from breaking wind and choking the jury.

Like it or not, memory loss hits the best and brightest. We lose our keys, forget where we stashed our purse, and have total brain-lock when it comes to meetings and appointments. "Huh," you'll think, "did I really tell my husband I'd meet him for lunch? What made me do that? I don't even like barbeque." My guess is, all you heard was the word "barbeque" over breakfast, and it probably sounded pretty good at that particular second. So you mumbled a groan of delight and your husband took that as his cue to make plans. While he rattles off the details of when and where, you're still dreaming of ribs, chicken, potato salad and peach cobbler, and miss the last part entirely. By the time lunch rolls around, you've already had two snacks, and you're currently fixated on the hamburger you saw on a billboard while heading to work. Well, call off the dogs; hamburgers are lunch today! As for barbeque, what on earth was your husband thinking?

Perhaps the scatterbrained nonsense is to prepare us for the stuff we'll miss once the baby arrives. Forget to brush your teeth? Oh well. Deodorant got missed this morning? Too bad (for everyone else). Hubby's favorite cola got passed up on the grocery store shelf? Cry me a river. And, oh yes, does that dermatologist appointment keep slipping your mind? I suppose that mole will have to grow some legs before we care.

Now, I know what you're thinking. "If I'm so forgetful, I'll surely forget my baby somewhere!" All new mothers fear sticking their infant's carrier on top of the car, loading groceries, and driving off without another thought. Here's the good news about that. It won't happen. Even if you're a walking zombie from lack of sleep, the baby will be your only focus, and you'll be on automatic pilot while taking care of your tooty-bug.

I really think that's why we forget everything else. We're too zoned on our little bundles to care who we're supposed to meet for lunch, how much dog poop piles up in the yard, or whether our husbands have clean underwear. But do you think we forget diapers, formula, wipes, burp rags, blankets, binkies, and five extra pairs of baby booties anytime we set foot out the door? Pul-ese!

You will eventually get back into the swing of a somewhat normal routine and be amazed at how much information you can juggle in a day. The (just slightly) bad news is that this usually takes a couple of years. Once you have kids, all priorities shift, all former routines are hacked, and all your focus goes to the care of the most important person on earth – your baby.

Most new parents are wound so tight for the first couple years that it takes that long to get all the knots out of the string. You'll relax a bit when you realize how resilient your child really is, but that won't be until she's falling off of every chair in the house, tripping and smacking her face every five minutes, and trying to eat each and every cricket she finds. When she survives these trials with nothing but minor boo-boos and a few howls, you'll be on to bigger and better worries – like remembering to call an exterminator.

Lack of Concentration: One of the things that men will never understand is the awesome miracle of actually growing a living being inside you. Knowing that cells are dividing and forming *a child* right inside of your belly is really just too overwhelming at times. Then, when that child starts to kick and squirm and change your body into a baby football field, well, that just tears it.

I recently went to my 20-week sonogram and still couldn't believe that a fully-formed, thumb-sucking baby was actually swimming around in my uterus. Three times around, and it still completely floors me that nature can do such a thing. Not only that, but technology allows you to see all chambers of that tiny heart, every moving finger and limb, fluid in the bladder, facial structure, and a whole host of other tee-nincy baby parts.

Now, what was my point? Oh yeah. Concentration. When you are making a human being with nothing more to start with than one single egg and a few persistent sperm, it can keep your mind going all day just marveling in wonder. Managing to get past the awe of conception only leaves you day dreaming about a perfect little nose, mouth, and tiny hands and feet.

As you progress in your pregnancy, the dreams and mind-wandering only intensify. Your body is constantly changing and reminding you of the big day ahead. The clock is ticking, and you've got baby-stuff to do! Preparing, pampering, and purchasing will consume all thoughts and concerns from here on out. It's no big surprise that you can focus on nothing but your impending birth.

You'll spend your days shopping for (or at least thinking about) baby supplies and maternity clothes. The nightly entertainment will include whipping out the belly and watching your little gymnast thump and contort your navel. Grabbing hubby's hand, you'll place it on your abdomen, and insist he feel this miracle he helped create. (He'll promptly get super-creeped-out when he feels something squirming in your stomach, but what can you expect? He's a guy.) Your spare time will be spent reading every single printed word on pregnancy and childbirth. When you finally fall asleep at night, your dreams will be laden with cribs, bottles, hospitals, and talking babies with beards. (We'll have to consult the experts on that one.)

Mind-boggling acts of nature aside, you'll eventually get used to being pregnant, and your concentration may switch focus to the minor (or major) irritating aspects of carrying a child. The physical toll of making a baby really takes shape in the last trimester, when thoughts are bent on simply getting a full night's sleep or ensuring nobody touches you in your general pissed-off state. The last month is especially trying and can transform the best of us into pit bulls. You are so ready to get that child out of your body that nothing else in life is more important, and heaven help the person who disagrees.

So whenever you get lost going to your mom's house, walk out the door with mismatched shoes, forget your jacket when it's snowing, leave your keys in your car, or accidentally bleach your husband's favorite pair of jeans, remember - it's all normal. You may feel like you're losing your mind, but your brain is just kicking out the unnecessary and making room for all the new concerns of the greatest joy and toughest job you'll ever have.

Chapter Four: Second Trimester Bliss

Hitting the second trimester is like walking onto a sunny beach after being frozen in the tundras of Russia. Your belly bloating fades, nausea subsides, prenatal vitamins make you positively zippy, and you begin to accept - and possibly even like - your changing form. Most women tell me they felt great during the second trimester. You have enough of a belly that you look pregnant, but you can still hide it if you want or manipulate your clothes to make yourself look adorable and glowing. You generally won't have gained enough weight (in the beginning anyway) to make you miserable, and you smile and giggle in response to every tumble and kick Jr. performs.

Unless you're one of those queen gestators that everyone hates, the second trimester is when you start to feel better, look better, eat better, and enjoy yourself immensely. Your little puff of a belly isn't quite big enough to cause tremendous discomfort, but it's obvious enough that you can start using it as an excuse to get the last seat at Christmas mass, cut in line at the grocery store, and make everyone scramble to ensure your comfort.

As with all things in life, there are a few little issues that might cause some bumps on your free-sailing sea, and of course, I'm the gal to warn you about any rough waters ahead. This chapter describes a few of the big changes you might encounter and wonder about. Medical reference guides tend to either scare mommies-to-be over nonsense issues or gloss over some big hairy deals, so we'll set the record straight here.

Enough with the Weight Already!
Beach Bound, Baby! (Weight Gain): I'm sure you've read this from no less than five other sources, but we'll go over it again in case you aren't quite a believer. If you've stayed within the recommended 0-4 pounds of weight gain for the first trimester, then you are free as a bird to gain about one pound a week from now until about four weeks from D-Day. When in your life have you ever been so open to indulge and enjoy

eating? Our whole life is spent counting calories, carbs, and fat grams trying to stay as trim and fit as a Playboy centerfold (just WHO the hell are we kidding?!) yet here we are, given the green light to gain and be happy!

The only problem with this liberation is that it's not as if we *can* gain that much weight *if* we want to. Little baby-to-be will make *sure* that we gain that weight - and then some - if we aren't careful. The food cravings and intense desire to eat everything in sight is so strong in the second trimester that it's freaking alarming.

My friend Amy and I aren't big eaters in general. However, when gestating, all bets are off. Food is a top priority. We happened to be pregnant at the same time with our last babies. While I claim amnesia on this one, she swears we once sat down with a bag of tortilla chips and a carton of plain Jane sour cream, moaning with pleasure through every last bite. Apparently, we even licked the bowl of sour cream clean and fought over who got the corn chip crumbs.

My advice in this department is to try not to gain too much weight too quickly. Spread out the thrill. Don't keep eating until you're miserable and waddling out the door of the deli. Try to limit the more terrible indulgences of fast food, candy, cake, ice cream, and other delicious fats to one tiny portion per day, or better yet, once every few days or once a week. I've heard the lame advice to satisfy your sugar cravings with fruit-sweetened cookies or applesauce (will someone PLEASE give me a break?!), but I live in the real world and that won't even begin to cut it. You can, however, try to stretch that sweet tooth by eating things like frozen yogurt, whipped cream with fruit (oooh, on angel food cake!), or granola with vanilla yogurt in between desperate forays to the cookie jar. They're still loaded with sugar, but they just don't sound as bad. Know what I mean?

If you believe everything you read, you may be scared to death of the sugar content in many of the foods previously considered "good". I've been told that bananas convert straight into sugar, fruit juices are about as horrible for you as a bottle of maple syrup, and granola is so loaded with sugar that it ranks close to "death wish." My personal take on fruit is that as long as it has very dark, rich, or bright colors, it's good. Melons, berries, apples, and pomegranates are my favorites.

As far as regular food goes, I've actually been beaten down enough with the processed foods hype to believe that any label listing "partially hydrogenated" *anything* is bad for you. Similarly, any food or drink with a sugar content over 10 grams per serving makes me wince. However, when pregnant, I tend to ignore my normally ingrained food philosophy and excuse anything edible that doesn't hurt my teeth when chewing. Where this leaves you, I have no idea, but at least you'll know that if you fall off the healthy food wagon, you're in fine company.

If you're having some trouble in the weight gain department and your doctor is worth the price of their fancy scrubs, they'll help you figure out what foods are best for you and how much you should actually be eating. It may take going to a dietician, but if the help is offered, take it. Food is a confusing subject. When you throw in the latest professional opinions on negative reactions to certain chow, sheesh. We'll just blubber a river of pregger angst.

For years now I've been avoiding white bread (with the exception of homemade cinnamon rolls – those don't count) and eating only whole grains under the assumption that grains are healthier than bleached white flour. Then along comes my mom, touting some book that says I shouldn't be eating wheat and grain because of my blood type. Apparently, my body will convert the food into some horrific chemical form, zapping me of energy and leaving me to die some miserable and convulsive early death. (Thanks Mom! Will do!) Okay, maybe I exaggerate, but you get my point. See a professional if you need to, and forget about trying to figure it out on your own.

Forever Fat: Will This Weight Ever Come Off? Alright girlfriend, you're a smart gal and you know just as well as I that after the baby is born, you can lose the excess weight. Even if you gained seventy pounds, it's entirely possible to eat right, exercise, get it off, and keep it off. If you've stayed within the recommended weight gain, then for the most part, you'll gradually shrink back down to some semblance of your former self without having to do too much starving or Pilates. Hips may stay spread a while. Things may be stretched and mutilated. And, unlike my miserably skinny sister (I say that with the most affection), you may not be able to squeeze into your favorite pair of jeans two days post partum. But your body will eventually (hopefully...okay, maybe not) tighten back up like saran wrap under a hair dryer. How long this will take varies greatly from person to person, but the standard six-week recovery time is not to be confused with how long it will take to be "you" again.

You've heard this a jillion times, but it takes nine long months to ripen a baby, and it will take at least that long to fully spring back. With the exception of my sister and my best friend, both of whom have some sort of genetic anomaly allowing them to melt back into their former selves in about a week, everyone else on the planet will need a good six weeks just to get their uterus back to normal - and another eight months or so to get rid of that last bit of unwanted fat.

You will probably still look pregnant two weeks after delivery (I HATE that), but if you consider how long it took your belly to balloon to its monstrous state, two or three weeks to shrink back down really isn't all that bad. Just be prepared for explanations when some blockhead doesn't see the baby carrier, stroller, and diaper bag you're lugging around and eagerly asks, "When's the baby due?" Yes, this has happened to me.

Did I Just Eat Fire? (Heartburn and Such)

Speaking of all this eating and ballooning, if you haven't experienced the joy of heartburn and indigestion yet, the second trimester is time to begin the love fest. Dreams of chicken wings, spicy Chinese, and onion rings keep you drooling all day, but if you happen to indulge, it'll also keep you gagging all night. Even your normal, everyday, healthy food choices will come back to haunt you as soon as your head hits the pillow. Those accursed hormones will relax the digestive tract valve that keeps food down, allowing that horrid acid to creep back up and set your chest on fire.

Solution? Well, I'm not about to suggest staying away from the fabulously spicy food, because that's just plain lunatic. But if you do dive in, go moderate. Don't eat until you're rolling, and try to make it early in the day or evening so you don't end up like my pregnant friend Lacy. An hour after wolfing a Greek dinner, she had her husband poised to dial 911. She was convinced this was it – death. Dead. Dying. Done. She had smartly taken a Zantac before dinner and another at midnight but was still gagging on acid. She miserably drank about a quart of Milk of Magnesia, gargled with salt water, and downed some ginger ale, but still couldn't lay flat without choking. She ended up trying to sleep propped on twelve pillows, but only managed to pinch a nerve in her neck. Being the loving and sympathetic friend I am, I peed my pants with giggles and told her she walked right in to that one. Granted, she tried to head off trouble, but if you are *planning* on a problem before you even start eating... Uuumm, yeah. Stupid.

So, avoid eating troublesome stuff within an hour or two of bedtime, and have a small glass of milk. I don't remember where I heard it, but I've been trying that lately and it seems to help. Keep some Maalox, Mylanta, Tums, or Milk of Magnesia handy and chug a little as necessary. Keep your head propped on at least two pillows. When you are miserably positive that acid is going to shoot out of your mouth and land all over your husband, get out of bed and try to relax upright in an easy chair. You still probably won't get much sleep, but those are the breaks. Sleep is a tough commodity when you're pregnant, and acid reflux is only one of the many reasons you'll spend much of the next few months tossing and turning. And cussing and crying.

As far as indigestion goes, good gravy. That nonsense sneaks up and knocks you silly. With my first kid, I couldn't handle chips and salsa (a staple in Texas, so this was not a good thing). Second kid, it was steak and horseradish. Go figure, if you gave me deviled eggs dipped in chipolte sauce or hot wings with ranch dressing, I'd be fine. But if one tenth of an ounce of horseradish got into my system, look out bathroom, here we come.

Pickled Asparagus with Marshmallows, NOW! (Speaking of Indigestion) The part of your noggin in charge of eating goes haywire, sending you reeling over fish smells one minute and running for chow mein with chocolate sauce the next. You'll crave and eat some of the most insane culinary concoctions you ever dreamed of. From raw potatoes and lemons to non-food items like ash and dirt, your brain will try to convince you to eat some mighty weird stuff.

When it comes to regular food items, as long as you're sure you won't puke after eating pickles dipped in marshmallow cream, have at it. In fact, the more disgusting the food, the better – that way hubby won't raid the pantry, leaving you in a rage the next time you reach for strawberry jelly and bananas. However, if you happen to crave non-food items, call your doctor immediately. It's very rare, but some women will actually crave really crazy things like coal, clay, cloth, or even turpentine. It sounds bizarre, but it has been known to happen, and obviously, you don't want to ingest these items!

Your cravings are on a rampage, but as far as the uber awesome, spicy, salty, yumm-o stuff, go easy until you know what sets you off. Pansy foods like grilled cheese sandwiches and tomato soup are usually safe. Test those waters when it comes to the delicious stuff; tummy tantrums are no fun. If you do end up in a lurch, you can simply avoid any more food or medicine until your belly stops screaming, or use those same old heartburn remedies to try and calm it down. Gooood luck.

And the Gas Goes Ever On (Fartle Hell): As the second trimester really gets going, the lovely sounds emanating from your body will continue to disturb and alarm you. In fact, it will probably be getting worse with the pressure of your growing baby. The thing about the gas is that it's not just about being physically uncomfortable. It's also about the people around you. You try so hard to be polite and save your colon blows for private places, but the gas of pregnancy doesn't always care. It sneaks up on you (fartle!), lets loose, and scares *you* just as much as it frightens the listener. Just last night, an obnoxious fart yanked me out of a perfectly sound slumber. My gracious husband claims not to have heard, but I'm sure he's lying to protect the precarious feelings of his bloated bride. Startled enough to shoot straight up in bed, I gasped in horror, "What was that?!" Yes, I was in a sleep-induced haze, but what else could it have been other than my own butt? Perhaps a goose had magically pecked its way into our home, wandered upstairs, and announced its presence by honking with ferver?

It's extremely disheartening to lose control of your keister and esophagus to the point that you can't stifle the embarrassing toots and burps. They just erupt out of your body in unpredictable increments and render you paralyzed with grief and mortification. It's enough to make you want to skip church, weddings, meetings, or any other event that doesn't involve enough chaos or noise to cover up the indecencies.

But look, if you happen to humiliate yourself, don't worry. Those of us on the empathy bus will gracefully ignore the interruption. Those who haven't yet been in your shoes will hopefully have enough decorum and etiquette to do the same. If there is a child or insufferable adult around who just can't resist ribbing and attempts to disgrace, take it in stride and calmly threaten to throw them to the ground, squat on their head, and fart them into being sorry.

Bursting Belly: To keep from feeling like you're going to explode when you're starving enough to consume an entire cow, eat small, frequent meals. In fact, just munch all day long. Keep the food healthy and light (lots of greens, veggies, and fruit) and it won't fill you up as much. Heavy, fatty foods will sit on your stomach longer and force you to walk around moaning in distress. Believe me, people stop sympathizing after a few weeks of stuffing your face with brownies. You'll get no moral support if you keep loading up like a dump truck and expecting people to listen to incessant griping, belching, and volcanic toots. Don't get me wrong. I'm right there with you in the hungry department. But I'm also a major complainer and I've learned that people (spouses in particular) get mighty annoyed when you eat like a horse then proceed to bitch and release obnoxious gas for the next three hours... or until all is digested and you're hungry again.

Fugly Veins and Sexy Swollen Woo-Woos

Varicose (Very Gross) Veins: A hugely hot topic of mine: varicose veins. The weight of your uterus can put some mighty pressure on your veins, causing them to bulge, deepen in color, or appear as rope-like appendages on your leg. It is no-shit unattractive, but the pain can be worse than the ugly. Luckily, it varies. Sometimes your feet will tingle or your legs will just be a bit achy by the end of the day. For people with horrid veins, the pain can be like fire running down your leg, crippling you into limping around and yelling in agony just as soon as you get out of bed each morning.

Having the worst varicose veins in all of gestating history, I've read all the lame advice concerning the care of them. I'm quite appalled at the lack of coverage this topic gets in pregnancy books. My second pregnancy produced a lovely rope-like vein on my right leg, running all the way from my disgustingly huge vulva (yes dear, you can get them there, too) to the bottom of my ankle. My doctor wrote me a prescription for some outrageously expensive medical support hose, and at the time, I had to go to an in-hospital medical supply store (please!) to get them. The compression needed to squeeze the circulation back into my legs called for hose so taut that heavy-duty household rubber gloves were the only way to even get a grip on them. THEN it took about five minutes just to tug, pull, and inch the blasted things on every day.

This third pregnancy has mashed my blood flow into double the horrific and excruciating veins all the way down my leg. Keeping with tradition, they're only on the right side and start at my love-bun. The ugliness is so bad that my doctor sent me to a vascular surgeon who was all too happy to suggest I go under the knife (while pregnant, thank you) to correct them. (Is everyone on the planet nuts or is it just me?)

Which brings us to treatment. Most of you need not worry that your veins will look or feel this bad. I've never met, or even heard, of anyone else with this much trouble (cue violins, please). Many times, if your legs are swollen and achy, all you need to do is ask your doctor about compression hose. Sometimes you can even get away with wearing regular hose, as long as they're thick and not sheer.

When talking about true medical compression hose, there are different grades of compression running from minimal to high. If this is your first foray into the joy of squeeze-puppies, you will need a professional assessment of the pressure appropriate for your legs, a measurement to get the correct size, and education on how to put them on. They're thick and tight, and you can't scrunch them up at the toe and ease them on like regular hose. There's an art to getting these monsters on, especially navigating a huge belly, and it's a colossal pain in the ass.

You can buy these hose online or at a variety of pharmacies or medical supply stores. Be prepared to pay hefty prices. They'll run anywhere from $50-150 for full support (not knee-high or thigh-high), and insurance doesn't always cover them. For my current pregnancy, since I knew what I was looking for, I was able to buy mine online at Healthylegs.com, and was most pleased with the service, help, and discounted prices. If you do buy them online, be sure to measure your legs exactly as they show you on the website and request the instructional video on how to put the hose on. If you need a high compression, you may need to invest in a pair of heavy rubber household cleaning gloves. Just make sure they have nice ridges on the fingers so you can get a grip on the hose. *Healthylegs* sent me a free pair of gloves, but they didn't grasp as well as the standard yellow household kind.

It's best to put the hose on *before* you get out of bed in the morning because as soon as you stand up, the circulation pressure makes the veins hurt and swell. I don't exactly follow this advice because (a) I have to pee within ten seconds of waking up, so it's bathroom first, legs be damned, and (b) I shower right after that. However, I usually flop back into bed once I'm clean and elevate my legs to shrink the fuglies down again before putting the hose on. I've also been known to crawl around my bedroom on all fours in an attempt to keep the pressure off until I get those stupid hose on. Wait, wait. Don't cuss the hose! Forgive me, hose. I love you and need you.

Speaking of, that's another way to reverse the pressure on your veins – lie or sit down and elevate your feet. Alternate sitting and standing during the day, as doing either for too long is hard on your legs. Lastly, and importantly, you will need to exercise those legs as your doctor permits (walking or swimming is probably best) to keep your circulation as healthy as possible.

As far as surgery, most doctors won't touch a pregnant woman's legs with a ten-foot pole. It's not exactly the safest thing in the world and often useless. The pressure of your uterus is the culprit to begin with. Until you give birth, there's no fixing that problem. Why my own vascular surgeon recommended surgery for me now, I'm sure I don't know. Maybe because he's a *surgeon* – that's what he does, but maybe my veins are just bad enough to warrant it. There is the possibility of the veins irreversibly discoloring my legs, not to mention the grace of a lovely purple-blue lump inside my thigh (caused by reversed blood flow) which he is concerned might clot and ulcerize. However, having discussed it with my OB, I'm willing to take the risk and wait until delivery. Ugly legs, here to stay!

Obviously, it would behoove us all to keep the weight gain within the recommended range so we can get back into shape quickly and keep unnecessary poundage off our veins. But beyond that, if we opt out of treatment, we'll just have to grab the doc and have her/him look at the fugly-wuglies during our first post-partum visit in the hospital. We can discuss options and go from there.

Varicose Vulvas – Good Gravy! That Actually Happens?! Lucky you, (and welcome to my world!) if you are cursed with varicosities on your vulva. There isn't a heck of a lot you can do to relieve the pain other than lying flat and/or compressing the veins with your hand or a folded or rolled washcloth. Sure, it's tacky as hell to go around clutching your crotch all the time, but how else are you supposed to get enough compression in that area and keep the swelling down? Full-length hose do help, but they aren't meant to compress the goodies. Just leave your ladylike hands off the woo-woo while in public. Once you get home, feel free to limp around, mashing and squashing all you want. If you're really desperate, go online and research the Fembrace V-Brace. It's a diaper-looking thing that's supposed to relieve the discomfort. At this point, I'll wear it on my head if it will help!

Captain Huge for the Rest of You! Warning for this section, ladies!! This does not happen to everyone – thank heavens for small favors. I certainly don't mean to scare you to death, so don't panic yet. I'm just saying, things may get dicey under the undies. Generalized vulvar engorgement is common and rears its ugly head in the second or third trimester.

Maybe, just maybe, you have escaped the joys of varicosities "down there". But lo! You may still get yours, indeed, my honey muffin! So let me introduce you to your basic, everyday, swollen love bun: it's rather like two lumpy bratwursts stuck between your legs. How on earth does it fit down there, you ask? Very tightly. (I feel sorry for the panties.) If you manage to get your mirror game going and take a gander, make sure you're near toilet paper. Not because you'll need it for goo (which you might), but to wipe your eyes when you start bawling and screaming. Intensely scary. I swear, sometimes my private parts get so lopsided and swollen that if they weren't attached to my body, I could NEVER i.d. them in a line up. The whole thing is engorged beyond recognition (really now, how well do you know your woo-woo?) and the blood-filled bluish-purple tinge makes you wonder if life is being utterly choked out down there.

With all this unyielding distention, one might think it will affect a vaginal delivery. Surely it will be impossible for any more stretching or enlargement! Ooh, girl. Sorry. Yes, you will stretch more, yes it will be revolting, and yes, a tiny human head can indeed get through. My swelling is about as horrid as it gets, and I delivered last time just fine. Your doctor will most likely keep an eye on it. If you are the slightest bit concerned, make sure to express those worries and keep an open dialogue with your caregiver.

And this brings us to the best part. After my last baby, it took all of about eight hours for that nasty swelling to disappear completely - varicose vulva and leg, engorgement - all of it. Many doctors and professionals may tell you that the vein problem will only get worse, but in my case, the only problem was the weight of my uterus. Yahoo! So if you happen to suffer with these ailments, here's to hoping your engorged goodies and varicose uglies will disappear after birth!

Grraaar! Tiger Stripes and Angry Skin

The second trimester marks the beginning of some serious weight gain, resulting in a quick expansion of your poor skin. I keep hearing all these wonderful stories about women who love the hormones of pregnancy because it provides lush and sheen to hair, nails, and skin. Personally, I've never met one of these ladies. Most women I've talked to have more complaints about their skin than anything nice to say. Between the bloating, baby, and plain old hormones, your delicate skin can get stretched, striped, blotted, and spotted beyond recognition.

The first pitfall is your face. Acne loves a pregnant woman's nose, chin, and forehead. Those blemishes must really think they're loved and welcome as much as they show up to decorate the most noticeable part of your body. You can scrub, exfoliate, moisturize, and nuke your face as much as you please, but those little babies still manage to pop up like a hateful cousin at a family reunion. Go ahead and care for your face by keeping it clean and treating spots, but don't expect any miracles.

You may also notice red splotches on your face called "chloasma." While unsightly, they should disappear after delivery. In the meantime you can try to cover them with a good foundation. Just be careful not to overdo the make-up and consult a professional on the correct color you need. Believe me, a red spot is less noticeable (especially to other tsk-tsking women) than heavy, miscolored make-up.

The most noted skin changes you will probably encounter are stretch marks and veins. Your boobs alone will get so huge and heavy that you might as well stick half a large cantaloupe into each side of your bra. Hands, feet, and face retain enough water to float you, and your belly looks like you swallowed a hot air balloon. With all this stretching and contorting, it's no wonder your skin holds a little protest in the form of red or white stretch marks and showy veins.

The stretch marks generally show up on your belly, sides, butt, legs, and possibly your exploding boobs (but hey, I think your fingers and toes are safe). Now, I've heard it go both ways on whether all those special creams and lotions keep the stripes at bay. My doctor and several friends refuse to believe, but other friends swear by it. It's very possible that it's all heredity, but who knows? Go ahead and use the creams if you feel like it. At the very least it will cut down on the dryness and excessive itching, which can make you wish you had talons. Speaking of, do your best to keep your claws off your belly or you'll end up with even more damage.

Therapy: My New BFF

If you haven't already guessed from all my moaning and complaining, the second trimester can bring on all sorts of aches and pains. I've already mentioned the muscle and ligament changes that accompany pregnancy. Your skeletal structure will also change, possibly causing some real discomfort. First of all, the weight of your belly will sometimes compel you to "let it go" and walk around with your stomach thrust forward. This creates a swayback, puts too much pressure on your spine, and causes back pain.

The second thing that can throw you around is the loosey-goosey movement of your pelvic bones. Due to pregnancy hormones, your entire pelvic region goes on a siesta in preparation for spreading during birth, and creates joints that jiggle and contort more than usual. This can cause some extreme pain, and in some cases (that would be pathetic little ol' me) occasionally render you immobilized.

I happen to be a huge believer in therapy for these nuisance pains. Deep tissue massage and physical therapy are intimate friends, but I would also whole-heartedly recommend Swedish massage, chiropractic care, yoga, spa treatments - you name it. If there is any way you can indulge yourself and splurge on these comforts, drop everything and make an appointment. In order to get physical therapy, you would probably need a doctor's order, but if you're in that much pain, you've most likely already discussed it with your caregiver.

There are also massage therapists who work on pregnant woman. Now, don't confuse *regular* massage with massage *therapy*, because they are two completely different things. The first time I went to massage therapy, I expected to be rubbed and relaxed and to generally just drift right out of the pain I was having in my arms and hands. Great balls of fire, was I shocked to tears. Message therapy is a *bear* because the therapist has to work all the kinks out of your tightened and mangled muscles. Car accidents, injuries, surgeries, and a host of other potshots to your body can seriously damage your muscles over your lifetime. You may not even notice this harmful accumulation until you go in to have those babies worked on. Holy moly, purple elephants and lighting bugs, it can be painsville galore, so be prepared.

Qualified, experienced, and *good* massage and physical therapists are absolutely worth their weight in gold. Although the therapy is sometimes uncomfortable at best, the long-term pain relief is immeasurable. Obviously, there are some quacks out there, so be careful in your choice. Get a personal or professional recommendation because these people should be highly trained to work on pregnant women. If you get one who doesn't know what they're doing, they can possibly inflict some serious damage. But if you find a good one, grab 'em!

If you're not in enough pain to warrant massage or physical therapy, go and get a regular massage, facial, manicure, pedicure, or whatever floats your boat. Pamper yourself if you're achy and uncomfortable. It will take your mind off your woes and make you feel better. Toward the end of the second trimester you'll be getting nice and plump, and if you aren't just delighted with your condition, you may need the distraction. Any therapy that helps you relax and enjoy your preggy-self is worth the price of admission.

DANGIT, I Need Some ZZZ's!

Once your belly starts rivaling a basketball, you'll begin to approach your sleep with insane protectiveness. Tossing, turning, gagging, choking, moaning and groaning are all very normal activities for the uncomfortably pregnant lady. My husband is so used to the exasperated sighs, shaking bed, burps, and farts, that I think he actually sleeps through most of it. Give your own hubby a month or two and he'll do just fine. If not, tell him to either get bent or go and sleep on the couch, because it'll only get worse before it gets better.

The first problem that begs attention is the fact that you can no longer sleep on your belly. This can be a huge source of anxiety for those of you used to hugging the mattress. I cannot even express the weeks of grieving and woe I endure before surrendering to my sides. Lord have mercy, I hate it, I hate it! Seriously, when is someone going to invent a King mattress with a hole in JUST the right pregnant-lady spot? Well, okay...not a good idea. Picture the lawsuits when pregger-Jane rolls on her back, gets her ass wedged in the hole, and does a pregnant-belly-split-leg jackknife. Not a pretty thought.

So. If we must be on our sides, the best way to get comfortable is to get a pillow, stick the bottom half between your legs and the top half under your belly to support your uterus. You wouldn't imagine that your hips have spread so much that there is an entire foot of space between your knees, but that's what it feels like. Plus, if not supported, your lounging uterus will pull the attached muscles, making your back ache even more than when you've been on your feet all day.

Sometimes a huge body pillow works well. It's long enough to go from your legs to your head, and it's quite like hugging a very squishy man. Sleeping on your back is also an option, but hells bells, that can be uncomfortable, not to mention the fussing you'll get from your doctor. Laying on your back puts all the weight of your belly onto your spine and can decrease good blood flow to the baby. So unless you're floating in a pool, the supine position is not one of much relief. If you must lie flat, it may help to prop your head with a couple of pillows and put another under your knees.

The second thing that keeps you awake is your little karate champion. Nighttime is playtime as far as many babies are concerned, and there isn't much to do inside your belly but loop, twirl, kick, and punch. While quite amusing at first, it soon begins to piss you off, making you spout obscenities or yell in the middle of the night. Tell your husband in advance of this possibility so that when you shout "Will you STOP that?!" or "Good grief, will you *please* cut that crap out!" he won't take offense and storm out the bedroom with a few choice words of his own. If the carnival in your belly is just too much to take, and changing positions doesn't help, try a rocking chair. Sometimes the repetitive movement will lull your little boxer off to sleep.

The next item on the no-sleep agenda is heartburn. We've been over the remedies, but I'm telling you my friend, sometimes the acid is still murder. If I stupidly forget to put my handy bottle of antacid on my bedside table, poor hubby is in for it. Flinging covers off in a rage and flopping around like a two-hundred pound fish in my effort to get out of bed, I stomp off to the nearest medicine cabinet and gulp down half the bottle of liquid chalk with a few infuriated and colorful metaphors blasted out between swallows. Any husband who can sleep through that racket is not only used to sleeping with a hugely pregnant woman, but is probably the type who can sleep through his own thunderous snores.

Plain old anxiety and excitement are other sure fire ways to upset your slumber. Sometimes you may have indulged in a bit too much caffeine before bed, and that can certainly keep you up and buzzing. But even without the stimulant, your mind will be racing a hundred miles an hour with what-if, I-need-to, I-should-have, and I-wonder. "What if my water breaks in public?" "I need to order that baby furniture." "I should have asked my doctor about these hemorrhoids!" "I wonder what labor will be like."

The questions and scenarios will dash around your mind like toddlers at a water park. But forget it girlfriend - attempts at sorting through the muddle will prove impossible. Instead, try to clear your mind and relax by drinking some warm milk, reading a boring book, or watching your husband mumble in his sleep. Whatever you do, don't start getting ticked off that he's actually sleeping peacefully and you're not. Believe me, you'll have plenty of time to get him back. Once baby arrives, claim exhaustion and make him get up in the middle of the night to rock little sweet-ums, deal with fits of gas, or change all the obnoxious diapers.

I (gasp) Can't (gasp) Breathe! Another jolly that keeps you awake and distressed is the inability to catch your breath. As your baby grows, you may sometimes feel like your lungs are being crushed to smithereens. You may also feel certain that you will be the first woman in history whose belly actually pops, leaving the medical community speechless. All this stretching, shoving, and mashing is due to your bulging uterus putting a ton of pressure on your lungs and tummy. Eating two bites of salad can extend your stomach a mere fraction, yet make you feel like a whale. Expanding your lungs is often a giant feat, making you positive you'll suffocate before the forty weeks are up.

For those of us less stout of heart and more whiny of mouth (I'm first in line), these maladies are quite insufferable. Until you have this baby and eliminate both ailments, you are doomed to endure with only two choices of relief. To take the pressure off your lungs, get down on all fours and let gravity drop the weight of the baby. Sometimes you can try to stretch your torso tall and straight, but frankly, I don't see much help in that. Most of us aren't yoga instructors and can't possibly contort and raise our ribcage enough to make a difference. Getting down on the floor and making like a doggie should give you some temporary relief and allow you to fully expand your lungs. The other remedy you can try for some breathing liberation is to bravely don a swimsuit and get yourself into a pool. See if the buoyancy helps lighten your load.

Get This Knife Out of My Leg! A crucial detail in the life of a gestating woman is the presence and management of leg cramps. I couldn't begin to explain the science of acid and muscles or the biology that actually sets those monster pains off, but I do know they hurt like a mo-foe. There are conflicting accounts, but I think the general consensus is that pointing your toes will initiate a calf cramp and send you thrashing about with a flurry of unintelligible grunts and howls. The pain is so powerful and searing that it leaves you unable to do much of anything except gasp for air and furiously point to your leg when your husband rushes in, ready to call an ambulance.

To avoid the torment, get used to flexing your foot. If you normally cat-stretch in bed before you get up in the morning or go to sleep at night, FLEX, don't point! Even if pointing your toes doesn't seem to bother you, get into the habit of flexing instead. It only takes one episode of intense suffering before you make it a point to remember. When you forget (it will happen) and the pain grabs you, try your best to flex your foot. If nothing else, use every ounce of your being and will power to stand up - that should flex it enough to help. Or, you could try to rub the cramp out. If your husband walks in and sees you grabbing your leg in pain, he'll think you've surely broken it in half. Try to choke out something along the lines of, "Cramp!" or "Rub!" so he won't faint or freak out before you've gotten some relief.

So alright. Body aches, gas, belching, and cramps aside, you are well on your way to having this baby! Get used to the lack of sleep and putting the needs of others first, as your life is now all about it! This baby hasn't arrived yet, but she has surely taken over your body, and as soon as she pops out, your heart will be twisted to mush. This is a good thing, girlfriend, and I say it with all good will. You will be more than happy to give up all sleep, eating, peeing, life and limb for this child, so don't fret. Just know that you're halfway there! Soon enough you'll breathe in that delicious newborn smell and roll over dead before you would change any of the challenges associated with getting her in your arms! (Sniff, sniff...hand me a Kleenex!)

Chapter Five: The Trouble with Clothes

With first babies, maternity clothes are usually a source of great delight. It's just too fun to go shopping for big-bellied shirts and proclaim to the world, "Look at me, I'm pregnant!" The stores are full of other pregnant women and even the sales people are usually pregnant or newly initiated moms. Everyone is genuinely excited for each other and eager to share all kinds of great stories. It's like one giant preggie party. There are even little "belly pillows" in the dressing room for you to stuff into your new pants to simulate how big you will get and estimate if the garment will still fit in three months. Sometimes the pillows even come in the shape of hearts with lace trim and sweet satin ribbon.

The biggest problem with maternity clothes is not the clothes themselves, but the fact that with first babies, you will desperately want to wear them, but your belly doesn't swell quite as fast as you'd like. This leaves you popping out of your normal clothes but falling out of maternity pants. And forget maternity tops just yet – they will come down to your knees and look more like a skinny muu-muu than a shirt.

By your second baby, the desperation to stay out of maternity wear is so great that you'll hang on to your normal clothes until you're busting out like a sausage. You'll try all kinds of tricks to stay in your normal jeans and chic skirts. Leaving pants unzipped and stretching a rubber band across the button hole is the first option. If you waited several years for this second baby, you may have forfeited all style in your maternity wardrobe, forcing you to look outrageously dated or faded if you choose to switch over to your boxed up maternity stash. This could leave you distressed enough to cut up your most darling "normal" pants, sew in a stretchy patch, and save yourself the money and tears that go along with shopping for new and trendy threads. Heck, by the time you'll be able to wear your "skinny" pants again, they'll probably be out of style anyway, so what's the big deal?

Sometimes you can be so bloated that maternity clothes will do just fine early on. My Poker friend Carey once showed up for our monthly gig looking quite "puffy" (to put it delicately) around the belly. We knew she was trying to get pregnant with her second baby, but she hadn't announced any big news, so the other girls held their tongues in check. Carey finally smiled and said, "Yes, stop looking at me like that - I AM pregnant." Amy let out a huge sigh of relief, pronouncing, "Man, I wasn't going to say anything, but... *damn*!" We had all just seen Carey the month before, and the change was rather dramatic – all due to bloating. She was happily lounging around in stretchy maternity pants and had no problems going from regular clothes straight into maternity.

By the end of the first trimester or possibly a few weeks into the second, you should be plumping up quite nicely. During this transition, finding clothes that aren't too tight or too big is a challenge. If you don't mind spending the money, most maternity shops will have clothes specifically for this time period. They are generally either made of a stretchy material or have a tummy pouch that expands just enough to let you breathe but not enough to get you through the entire pregnancy. Girlfriend, get the stretchy kind because you can continue to wear your regular shirts with them. If you get pants with a pouch, you'll have to be creative in finding non-maternity shirts that are long enough to cover the pouch, but not so bulky that they fall off your shoulders and give everyone a free show every time you bend or lift up your arms.

The other option is sticking with non-maternity pants and simply wearing them below the belly. Depending on the current style, you may get lucky and be pregnant during a "hippie" year, when stylish pants are cut low on the hips. And, you may be able to get away with continuing to wear your cute little tees and sporty shirts with these pants. The shirts may start to hike up a bit and reveal the bump, but if you have a body worthy of show, go for it. However, if you aren't comfortable trying to imitate Hollywood fashion, go ahead and wear the chic pants - just start raiding Hubby's closet for shirts long enough to cover you up.

You could also head to the mall and try to find some shirts that are one size bigger than you normally wear. This allows some extra length, but not so much material up top that they look ridiculous.

The best route is to call up all your Mommy girlfriends and ask for any volunteers for a clothes dump. But don't be surprised if you find that newer Mommies aren't always thrilled to share their clothes. It's really quite understandable, so hold off on any scoffing. Maternity clothes, especially the really trendy and adorable kind, are expensive. If your friend has just spent an arm and a leg on a fashionable new wardrobe, even if she isn't wearing the clothes anymore, she may still be reluctant to hand them over quite so soon.

One thing you may not know, as Mommy-chic does, is that maternity clothes get some serious wear and tear. First of all, your pregnant breasts may leak, soaking every shirt you wear, possibly staining them with a leopard print of colostrum. Second, the butterfingers who wear these borrowed clothes tend to spill at least one teaspoon of every single dish they eat onto themselves. I kid you not, you will be shocked to see how many crumbs and blobs of mustard, ketchup, dressing, oil, and coffee end up on your clothes at the end of the day. Not only that, but you will wash and wear the same dadgum shirt so many times that it resembles a rag by the time you have the baby. So don't expect your friends to graciously hand over their maternity digs.

That said, if you happen to have very giving and generous buddies, feel free to jump with glee when they plop down fifty pounds of material for you to sift through. Sometimes you hit paydirt, but not always. When they have an older kid or two and joyfully pronounce, "Take it all – I never want to see it again as long as I live!" then that probably means the stuff is old, dated, and not very usable. They probably won't feel bad if they never actually see you wearing it, but just the same, you may want to pick out the stuff you might wear and respectfully ask them again if they'd like the rest back (before you throw it all in the fireplace).

The other problem with borrowing clothes is size. I have only one friend from whom I can borrow clothes, and even then, she's so tall that I often have to do some fancy pinning or sewing to get things to fit correctly. The rest of my friends come in so many shapes, sizes, and heights that there's really no use in even asking. Besides, it's too depressing to try on someone else's clothes and realize that they're too small, too long, or too tight across the chest. I'd rather go to a department store where I can curse a manufacturer or some cutesy pregnant model on a poster instead of my sweet friends who consistently lie and tell me I look so thin (bless those ladies!).

Where Do I Begin? All this "do I borrow/do I not" business can leave a girl depressed and confused. Is it really necessary to buy an entire new wardrobe of clothes that you will only wear for six months or so? On the other hand, is it actually okay to borrow someone else's clothes and beat them to smithereens? The only other option is to start raiding hubby's closet, but depending on the fashion trend of the day, you might end up looking offensive at worst, foolish at best. I've read all the advice to borrow your husband's pants, but for many people, that's just not feasible. My personal preference is to waddle around in my husband's sweats most of the time. I don't work right now, so the non-respectable hobo look is just peachy with me. I'm also not the type who gives much of a hoot what others think. I'm fat and depressed, so everyone else can like it or lump it – I don't really give a shit.

There are, however, working class gals and those who care a bit more about their appearance. Are you really supposed to show up at a business meeting or doctor's appointment wearing your husband's trousers? Some women borrow hubby's jeans, but frankly, I've had only one friend pull this off with style. The rest of us have quite a hard time. The pants may actually fit around the waist, but the legs just drag the floor and balloon out like a parachute.

The Preggie Bra

I think we've officially decided that unless you have rich and generous friends, you will need to head to the mall. The first item on the need-to-get agenda is, of course, a bra. Girly, don't even try to borrow these from your friends. Insanely desperate and shopping averse in general, I did just that, and oh, mistake! At first all was well and good, but it turned sour quick. Feeling so fabulous that I finally had some cloth to holster my monsters, I was crestfallen when Mr. and Mrs. Booby literally started busting out of those borrowed boulder holders in about two weeks flat – and I don't mean just busting out in the front. They were actually coming unhooked in the back!

I either had to stop wearing them or chance letting the dogs out in public. I can only imagine being forced to excuse myself to run to the bathroom with the angry beasts doing a rattle-jiggle dance behind my shirt. You think I'm joking about the horror of the Big Girls coming out to play, but the person I borrowed these bras from was the one Poker Mom who was gleefully ridiculed because her boobs were so outrageously huge when pregnant. It was just too comical and freakish for the rest of us to ignore! She's the only one in the group who was forced to find out what comes *after* "DD" in the bra alphabet. Busting out of *her* bras was bury-your-face-in-chocolate depressing.

We've talked a little about bras in Chapter 2, so we won't rehash here. Just remember that when you go to try them on, keep in mind that you may keep getting bigger throughout your pregnancy, so leave some room for expansion. Make sure the cup fits over your entire breast (nothing like a little cleavage on a nice rotund woman), and if you get an underwire, make sure it comes all the way underneath your armpit and grabs any stray boobie trying to escape. Also, you may want to keep in mind whether you plan to breastfeed or not. Many times you can go ahead and start experimenting with the breastfeeding bras to see which kinds are most comfortable for you. Some will even have hooks or notches in the front at the top so you can adjust to accommodate the changing size of your milk jugs.

The last order of business when it comes to bras is cleaning. Leaky breasts are often a source of embarrassment and frustration to new moms. Not only must you bear the horror of soaking your shirt at a fancy dinner party, but you must also deal with cleaning the darn things every time you turn around. You can, as one of my friends did, buy a gazillion and throw them in the washing machine as needed, but they won't last very long with all the ringing and twisting. At about twenty bucks or more for your basic bra, that can be an expensive time saver.

Go ahead and throw them in the wash if you so desire, but buy a cheaper variety and stick them in a mesh bag on a gentle cycle. If you want to invest in some better quality bras (highly advised!), buy two or three and hand wash them. I guess the price difference would even out if you wanted to buy more of them cheaply, but comfort is also key when you're pregnant. You'll have way too many other BS discomforts to deal with as you get bigger. There's no need to add to your misery with a crappy bra.

You can also save money and cleaning time by buying some nursing pads to stick in your bra. These are simply disposable, round, flat pieces of cotton that you put over your nipple to catch any small leaks and save your bra from stains. Look for them in the baby section of your favorite local store. They will usually be with the bottles and nursing accessories. These pads are little, so they may not catch enough to save your bra and self-esteem, but they should help.

The last line of defense is an actual plastic cup that you stick over your nipples to catch those vagrant ounces of fluid. You probably won't need something this dramatic until you are a full-fledged milking machine, but if you leak a great deal now, these cups are actually quite nifty. They do take up a lot of space, so be prepared to give up all sense of modesty – and buy an even bigger bra. Thank heavens I haven't needed to lay eyes on a pair of these cups in quite a while, but if memory serves, they also have a small air hole at the top. This means that, in addition to having to tote around a couple of loaded machine guns, you won't be able to bend over for any reason. Otherwise your stash of liquid may pour out the top and splatter all over your face. Just a thought.

Must I Really Wear Hippo Panties?

Good news on this front, my friends. You need not compromise your groovy sense of style for a pair of panties that reach halfway up your torso and allow your boobs to rest on the elastic. No, there are plenty of under-the-belly panties that will cover your ample booty just fine. In fact, you can even go for thongs. Yes, you can! You'll probably need a sumu size, but if they hide enough up front and you don't mind the constant wedgie and cheesy cheek show, go for it.

A sad fact of life is that pregnancy hormones will cause your woo-woo and rear end to swell in mammoth proportions, forcing you to buy a size up (or two - or four) in any regular panty you buy. I never understood why a woman's ass must distend along with her belly, but it seems that the human body can't take all that weight up front and must balance it out somehow.

Maternity underwear happens to be one of my favorite things in life. Aaaahhh! Freedom! Relief! Give it up and put 'em on, girl. Of course, you can always wait until your regular panties are so tight that half your rear hangs out the back. Or thongs cut into your hips like a blade, thus making a couple of rounds of flesh split down the middle...hey, something resembling MORE ass cheeks! In your desperation to deny your changing figure, you might cling to your sexy underwear like adhesive, but you'll only make your hiney look like it's being shoved into something it shouldn't.

Try to buy an under-the-belly style, in your normal, pre-pregnancy size, and they'll stretch, move, and grow with you. They're so wonderful that you can forget about strangulation, migration, or humiliation. What's even better, they're relatively cheap. I have about ten pairs that I paid seven dollars each for. These cotton beauties have made it through all three of my pregnancies. Currently in virtual tatters from overuse, I still proudly and lovingly put them on every morning. Buying more is not out of the question, but these guys are old and I've been unable to find the exact style elsewhere. Being my faithful self, I haven't strayed from my devotion and bought a different style yet. But if I did, I'm sure they'd be just as comfy.

Preggie panties should go with the flow of fashion. That being the case, the fit, design, and material will generally be comparable to the most popular undies you'd find at any old department store. Since fashion changes slightly from year to year, maternity underwear thankfully follows suit, and you shouldn't be stuck wearing something new, yet ugly and dated. You also need not worry about paying an arm and a leg for your skivies. Like every other article of clothing, prices will vary depending on where you purchase them. My advice is to go to a maternity store, buy one or two pairs and see how you like them. Then decide whether or not you want more of the same, a different style, or a knock-off from somewhere else. Keep in mind, expensive stores will carry expensive panties, so if you want something less pricey, don't head straight to the nearest affluent specialty shop.

The Basic Bored-Robe (um, I Mean Wardrobe)

Pants: After bras and undies, pants are the next priority. In the beginning, it's not so much that your belly swells and pokes out. Rather, you just get *round*. You waist disappears first, then the bootie starts to shoot out. Being unlucky in the bloating department can definitely cause some problems, but many times it's just a matter of spreading and puffing. You won't get that nice, perfectly spherical ball in your belly until the second trimester. (After your boobs and keister formally announce the arrival.) This makes finding pants a challenge. As mentioned earlier, it's best to try and find some transitional pants with a stretchy belly, not pants with a pouch. They will allow you to breathe and cease your worries of popping threads and ripping material each time you exhale.

As you get big enough to graduate into full-fledged maternity pants , you will definitely need the kind with a pouch, or the kind that are specific to the last months of pregnancy. They will be bigger in the bum and have ample belly space. If you try to buy these pants too early, it's difficult to determine how much space you'll need and what size. Holding them up and eye-balling a guess is futile. You will ALWAYS chink them back on the rack with confidence and snort, "Good gawd, my ass will NEVER be that big!"

Oh contraire, my dear. Go ahead and try them on – you may be surprised at how much gap you fill. Stuff the maternity pillows in there to gauge the future fit, but understand, it's not an exact science. You will never get a true sense of how tight the pants will be across your belly and rear until you are ripe with child and squeeze in that ballooning flesh. Unless they run large or small, most of the time you can simply buy your pre-pregnancy size and they will end up fitting just fine. Well, that is, unless we get ice cream happy and pack on a few extra (50) pounds.

My advice is to buy these pants only as you need them. By the end of the second trimester, you should have a good idea of how big you'll get. If you can either roll the top once or stick your hand in the pouch and extend it a good four more inches, you're doing well. Just allow for some liberal breathing room.

Still not convinced? Honey, the last month of pregger-land is killer. Your belly distends to proportions you wouldn't believe. (And if it doesn't, I do NOT want to hear from you, you skinny, rotten playboy barbie!) Believe it or not, you will want pants that stretch way beyond anything you dreamed you'd ever need. I scrutinized my biggest pair of maternity pants last night - and was astounded that they actually fit quite nicely. GREAT balls of fire, I'm still in my second trimester, and these were the babies that saw me through week 39 the last time around! FREAK-ing depressing. Now I must venture forth and bravely purchase yet more pants I'm sure I'll "never need." Uh!

Shirts: Transition shirts need some flexibility. You can certainly dig into your husband's closet for these, but I wouldn't recommend it unless you have a similar frame. Otherwise the shirt will simply hang on you screaming, "I don't belong here!" When trying to find a mate for stretchy pants without a pouch – well, here's the thing. There's a balance to achieve, girlfriend. Listen, I know you're trendy and love fashion – but let's not cling to the old self, shall we? At least not to the point where you refuse to put on anything that doesn't wrap you like saran. Cute little bodies can certainly throw on a long, tight shirt and go for it, but really...how many of us fit in that category? Seriously.

Don't ignore the mirror and insist on squeezing into shirts that hug the fat rolls. EMBRACE your bigger, beautiful self, girl! Buy some bigger shirts! Just one or two sizes bigger than you'd normally wear, I swear. This should give some extra length to cover any bulge and give you room to move. And don't get them so big up top that they fall off your shoulders and make you look like you've been swallowed by Mommy's dress-up clothes.

When the belly gets big enough that regular shirts (no matter what size) are too short and make you look dumpy, move on to "the tents." It's actually quite nice when you put on one of those maternity shirts and realize how much better they fit than regular shirts. As big as they are, once you get them on, the sheer comfort and freedom makes you sing. Laaaaa! It looks and feels so much better when the top half fits the way a shirt is supposed to and the bottom half attractively drapes and clings to your belly just enough to cover pouches and any rolly pollies you might find unpleasant.

Dress Clothes: I showed up for my last doctor's appointment looking all spiffed-up in my jeans and cotton t-shirt. Trend-a-roo! (Although keep in mind, when I take off my sweat pants and put on anything else, I'm spiffed-up.) As soon as I plopped my sorry self down on the couch in the waiting room, I spied a handsome couple doing their best to look occupied as they threw surreptitious glances at the rest of us sloppy pregnant women.

Being my nosey check-out-the-other-pregnant-women self, I boldly stared and took in every detail of the gestating woman's appearance. She had on a fabulous pair of black pants, boots, and a stiff white, crisply clean button-down shirt. It made me wonder, does she have a job that she has to head right back to, or do she and her husband just normally go around looking like they're headed to the Dallas Museum of Art and a lunch date with the Mayor? Not that I'm jealous, mind you. I'm far too lazy to bother getting that dressed up just to strip off my clothes and have someone shove a hand up my peanut checking for dilation. I am, however, just casually aware that I could look a lot less shabby and homeless if I invested the time and money into some nice threads.

Which brings us to you. Working gals and those who are more conscious of their appearance (again, I consider anything other than pajamas and work-out gear "conscious") will want to invest a little more in maternity dresses, suits, and professional wear. Even those of us who hate to bear our legs or put on anything that must be ironed should have at least three or four good ensembles in the closet. We will all obviously have church (YES, my potty mouth goes to church!), meetings, parties, and other events that call for us to ditch the comfy oversized shirts and put on something a little more respectable. And having one outfit is not enough, as you will end up wearing it so much that you'll want it doused with gasoline and burned by the time you hit your last month.

No lectures here on what to buy in the professional department, because I'm sure you can figure it out. But there is one last piece of advice for hot weather. If you're nice and big during the summer months, this is where sundresses come in extra handy. Not only are they cool, but so roomy and comfortable that you'll never want to take them off. Buy one or two short ones for casual parties, a day out shopping, or hitting a restaurant with a friend. In addition, get two or three long ones for work or more formal events that don't require hose. You may also need one nice formal dress - although personally, I'd wait until I was staring the necessitating event in the face before I went and bought one. If you get one "just in case," you simply won't know how the piece will fit with a monstrous belly. However, if it's on sale, roomy, and looks suitable, go ahead and buy it. Even if you outgrow it, chances are you'll use it at least once or twice before then.

Shoes (and Just HOW Do We Put These On?)

Shoes for the pregnant lady... Where do we begin? With slip-ons and flip-flops, of course. For casual wear, these shoes are absolutely invaluable. Once you hit the third trimester, bending over to buckle, tie, or pull on straps will be a source of raging screams and tears. Maneuvering around a huge belly to put on shoes is one of the biggest hassles in the life of a gestating lady. You can't sit on the floor to do it, because you won't be able to get up. You can't do it while standing because you'll lose your balance and fall flat on your face. And you can't sit on the bed or you'll get lost in the squishy mattress and have to call a couple of firemen for help getting off.

The key lies in finding a stable sitting surface that's just the right height for sitting. Spread your legs like you've got a cello between them. Then bend over to perform the task quickly before all the blood rushes to your head and starts gushing out your nose. You could also try to yank up one ankle and rest it on the opposite knee, but unless you've got muscles like a yogini, your ankle could just shoot forward in a loud protest that it's not supposed to be there.

Slip-ons and flip-flops allow you to remain standing, keep your head clear of congestion, and actually get your shoes on in less than five minutes. However, be forewarned, as I am talking only about slip on sneakers, sandals, or plain, flat, flip-flops. This does not apply to anything with a heel. Heels are not recommended *at all* during pregnancy, especially slip-on heels. Waddling around with cute and uncomfortable heels, especially if you can trip right out of them, is never a good idea. Having said that, I must confess that I just bought a pair of tight-toed, dreadfully painful slip-on heels. Why? I need them to go with the outfit I just bought to wear to a writing conference. Fully conceding my stupidity, and sheepishly accepting my friend's "you have no business wearing those shoes" comment, I'm sure I'll pay dearly. Moral of the story: Do as I say, not as I do.

If you can't manage to piddle around in nice, cushy slip-ons all day, wear shoes that are sensible, flat, and supportive. If you don't already have some in your closet, spend the extra money to get one or two pairs that you can wear to work and other non-trashy-shoe events. While you can certainly purchase knock-off shoes that are affordable and attractive, if you go cheap, they may still be unbearably painful. Not to say that expensive shoes aren't agonizing to your tootsies, but rather, cheap shoes *usually* are. Although, here again, I just found a pair of slip-on sneakers for $20 that made my feet feel like they were wrapped in pillows. Did I buy them? Of course not. I guilted myself out of the purchase and limped out of the store wearing my old, grungy, worn-out, ugly, no-support-to-your-aching-back slip-on tennies. If my husband knew this he'd probably throw a fit, as *he* is the one who has to pay for my discomfort. The poor guy graciously listens to all the moaning and griping about my sore back, achy muscles, and twisted spine. He'd gladly throw as much money my way as needed just to shut me up.

If I haven't already talked you into splurging a bit and getting some practical and comfortable shoes, remember that you'll be carrying around an extra thirty to fifty pounds by the end. AND your feet may be so swollen that squeezing them into anything with a closed toe may be out of the question anyway. Take my advice, learn from my needless suffering, and get yourself the shoes you need to be comfortable. Buy a size up or extra wide if the tootsies are too big for your current shoe stash. Don't worry about looking good, because nobody really expects a pregnant lady to walk around looking like a beauty queen. Besides, most focus will be on your belly, so allow yourself the freedom to wear butt ugly shoes – as long as your feet and back muscles love them.

Swimsuit Woes

Ooooh, touchy subject. I would highly advise swimming for recreation or sport no matter what the season. But if you cringe at the thought of showing the world your half-naked preggie self, you've got an uphill climb. Hopping on the weight or cardiovascular equipment at the gym may be out for you due to medical, financial, time, or laziness reasons (hey, no judging here). However, a pool is something that might actually be enjoyable to the full-bellied person and worth the extra effort.

My experience with pools and swimsuits has afforded me two very valuable lessons. First of all, adults generally tend to grin with sweet delight upon seeing a pregnant woman wade herself into a pool. You will get comments like, "Oh, that's so good for the baby!" or "You keep that up, honey. You're doing great!" Men and women alike always offer encouraging smiles and kudos.

Kids, on the other hand, are a different story. Those little mongrels will stare, gawk, and ogle with blatant amazement and curiosity. You can literally glare a hole in their head attempting to impose some sense of social etiquette and force an averted gaze, but it won't work. They're oblivious to all elbows in the ribs or parents hissing, "Stop staring!" What makes it truly ghastly is if you realize all the gaping is because your suit is falling off or leaving nothing to the imagination.

As luck would have it, my first pregnancy had me boasting my biggest belly during the hottest summer months here in Texas. As soon as the temperature started to notch above ninety, I headed straight to the nearest maternity shop for a swimsuit. Oooo, was I excited when I noticed they were on sale! Hastily waddling to the rack, I eagerly pushed hangers right and left to see what goodies I would find. My excitement soon turned to disgust as I realized the reason for the sale. The suits came in only two varieties: huge and ugly.

The price being right, and me being daring, I chose ugly and purchased my hot pink suit for all of seven dollars. Retrospectively, I think my morale was given a boost when another woman in the same dilemma (also stupidly buying the hot pink suit) gave me an understanding look and said, "Shoot, for seven dollars, I suppose we can't go too wrong, huh?" At the time, I agreed it was worth the gamble, but MERCIFUL HEAVEN! After wearing the suit on all of two occasions, I was mortified to learn how costly that seven-dollar mistake was.

The first go around braving the suit was to a public pool. I'm not sure how long it took me to notice the stares, but my first indication was, of course, some obnoxious kid watching me like I was a two-headed monkey. What on earth was his problem? Sheesh, I know I was big, but heavens, hadn't he ever seen a pregnant woman before? Since I couldn't very well yell at him to go find some manners, I simply lowered myself into the kiddie pool and pretended to be absorbed in the task of entertaining my friend's baby. As soon as I could, I jumped out of the pool and swiftly wrapped myself in a huge white towel. There. No more staring for you, young man!

I hopped in my car and raced home, wondering all the while if I was gushing blood, sprouting feathers, or had snot all over my nose. What on earth was that kid staring at? As soon as I took my towel off, I forgot all about my appearance. The towel was covered with so much pink dye that it looked like a flamingo had thrown up. So perhaps that was it. I was oozing pink whenever I moved an inch in the pool. Oh well. I vowed to use a dark towel next time and washed the suit in preparation.

Several days later my husband and I suited up and headed to the gym together. Once in the pool area, I cautiously disrobed and lowered myself into the water, glancing around to catch any giggles, pointing, or inappropriate gazing. The only stare I caught was my husband as he gasped, "Holy s@$#, honey! You can see right through that suit!" Apparently, the material lent itself to showing off my pancake size nipples, ample butt crack, and overgrown pubic hair. Just lovely! Well, at least the mystery was solved. (That poor kid will have nightmares for life.) So the next time we see a hot pink suit on sale for seven bucks, what do we do, class? Let's say it altogether, now... *"Run!"*

For the second go-round in the bathing suit search, I went straight to the high-priced maternity stores in the richest areas of town to find a suit that wouldn't fall off, look stupid, or entertain a crowd of onlookers. I found exactly what I was looking for in an elegant raised print, black one-piece. It was eighty dollars and I gladly forked over the cash so I could save what was left of my dignity. My advice to you is to do the same. As small a piece of clothing as it is, it's the one thing that can really make or break our self-esteem. If you get something cheap, then decide you don't like it and won't wear it, what's the point?

Maternity suits are slightly less depressing to shop for than regular swimsuits because, at the very least, you have an excuse for your outrageous knockers and dimply butt. With more and more people strutting around showing off their bellies, there is now a much better variety of styles to choose from. Maternity swimwear comes in one or two-piece, sporty, floral, classic, or sexy. You can also always get a nice wrap to go with it, which will successfully cover any cellulite or ghastly need for a pubic wax. It may cost a pretty penny, but if it motivates you to get out there and exercise, do it. Go ahead and splurge on a swimsuit. It will feel better, look better, and wear better.

Shhh! It's a Secret!

I've gone on and on about borrowing, buying, and binging on clothes, but what I haven't said yet could be the most important. Yes, it's highly likely that you'll need to spend money on at least some of your pregnancy wardrobe. But one thing that I have discovered only with this last pregnancy is that you can get great clothes, cheap. I happened to be browsing in a second-hand shop for kids when I spied the maternity wear. Drawing me like a magnet, I immediately started perusing. Not only did I find quality clothes from the expensive maternity shops, but they were so affordable that I nearly leaped with glee. Happy dance!

If you live in a relatively big city, there should be at least one or two second-hand shops in the richy froo-froo area. Find one for kids that sells clothes, furniture, and toys. Call or visit to see if they also sell maternity clothes. You can easily get an entire outfit that looks and feels great for a fraction of the cost of a brand name maternity store. In fact, the last time I was checking prices I hit a sale. The pricey brand name clothes were running about $10 for pants or shirts. Talk about your "Woo-hoo!" moment! I bought a beautiful red top, wore it home, and promptly ate a salad, splattering balsamic vingarette dressing all over the front. Did I care? Ha! At ten bucks, you can laugh at the stain. I can't imagine how I got a shirt in such great condition when I managed to taint it in a matter of hours, but whatever. People actually buy these clothes at regular prices from regular stores then proceed to wear them only once or twice. Yesssss!!

Now, the *kids* clothes at these second-hand shops don't always measure down to my el-cheapo price preference, but they are generally adorable, gently used or new, and well worth the money. The same goes for the maternity digs. In fact, they are usually cheaper because they don't sell as quickly. The greatest part is that you won't be subjected to sifting through dated and ugly clothes because these shops won't put them out to sell. If the store is located in a somewhat wealthy area, you need not worry that you'll look like a degenerate sorting through used clothes. The people buying (and selling) them are the same people that live in the area. You know how the best garage sales are the ones in uppity neighborhoods? The same principle applies to these second-hand shops. The merchandise they sell is basically new and in excellent condition. So hold your head high, get excited, and shop away – I promise I won't tell!

Chapter Six: Doctor Visits
The Good, The Bad, and The Ugly

Obstetrical visits can be a source of great joy. They can also be damn
dreadful. First of all, you have to get weighed and pee in a cup every
single time you step foot in the door. And you never know when you'll
have to strip down and be humiliated while the doctors and nurses
merrily go about their business. Sometimes they even have the gall to
start chatting away about vacations, weather, or your cute socks while
they've got you spread eagle with a hand or instrument up your crotch.
By the time you finish your OB visits, you'll have a much greater
appreciation of the gestating process. You will also have little or no
sense of pride left. But you *will* be (at least somewhat) prepared for any
unpleasant aspects of childbirth – like having twelve strangers march
into your hospital room just as soon as you start squirting bodily fluids
and pooping on the table.

Speak Up or Shut Up (You as the Patient)

Before we get too deep into doctor visits, we need to establish what
type of patient you are. We've talked about finding the right caregiver
for your personality and needs, but you also need to know how to get
the best care once you've picked a winner. Doctors and midwives are
not God. They are not infallible, consistently happy, and always willing
to indulge your every teeny-tiny concern or problem. Sometimes they
have bad days. They could be sick, or having personal problems, or
have been up all night delivering a baby – who knows. Given that, it's
best to look at how much handholding you'll need and how well your
particular caregiver can dole it out.

You have to remember that more questions pop up as your belly starts
popping out. Are you bold enough to ask them or are you too afraid to
"bother" your doctor with it? On the other side of the coin, are you
rolling into your appointments with a list of thirty questions and keeping
your doctor tied up for an hour? There is a balance to getting good care

by being a "good patient." Sometimes you can land a wonderful doctor and be just thrilled with their bedside manner, care, concern, and individual attention. This is ideal, as you need to feel comfortable and secure in their care. However, if you end up being too shy to talk about your concerns or hound them with a ridiculous list of "My nails are growing so fast – can you recommend a good manicurist?" questions, they are going to feel like throwing your big butt out the door.

First of all, your care is ultimately *your* responsibility. When you have a legitimate concern or question, ask. That is what your doctor is there for. When you're too afraid to ask, try to research it yourself first. Check all your books, online, or call the OB nurse coordinator if your caregiver has one. You must consider that this is your care, you are paying for it, and you deserve a satisfactory answer. Ask. If you end up disappointed because you couldn't find out the answer to something important to you, it's your own darn fault. Doctors are not mind readers, and they will not be able to help if you don't communicate.

At the other end of the spectrum, since your care is indeed your responsibility, do your doctor a favor and don't bombard him with a thousand stupid questions each time he enters the exam room. Take the same route as the mousy patient. Try to research the answers before you dump a bunch of irrelevant problems on your caregiver's lap. They will be more than happy to help you with any reasonable concerns, but don't keep them tied up over things like maternity clothes, your mother's harsh comments about the color of the nursery, and how to tell your husband that he's not the one who's pregnant and should stop eating so much. Not only do you hold up the doctor's care of other patients, you will begin to make them dread seeing you. Doctors are only human and will start reacting to your endless questions with quicker answers, drooping enthusiasm, and less genuine concern for you.

Don't Be a Toot: If you are irritating, whiny, obstinate, demanding, or overbearing (pul-eze, girlfriend, don't pull that crap!), you will both suffer in the relationship. Don't get me wrong, because at eight-months pregnant, I'm about as whiny, obstinate, demanding and overbearing as they come, but I *really* try to keep it in check when I'm at the doctor's office. In fact, I like to try and bribe the staff with cookies, muffins, and other baked goodies, just to make them look forward to seeing me. Hey, you catch more flies with honey.

During one of my physical therapy sessions, I met a nurse who worked in labor and delivery at one of the area hospitals. Trapped in the exercise room doing our daily reps, we struck up a conversation. Having worked at a hospital as a speech therapist, I've always known about the "bad patient" syndrome. There are just some patients you dread working with because they are flat out unpleasant, cranky, demanding, and rude. This nurse confirmed everything I've ever believed about nurses in labor and delivery – that as a patient, you need to be nice. The particular hospital this woman worked at was in a rather affluent area. Her bias wasn't against the amount of money these patients waddled in with, but the amount of special treatment they expected simply "because."

Her assessment was that most patients are fine, some were great, and a few are downright spoiled rotten and ugly. They whine about the beds. They complain about the pillows. They are too cold one moment, too hot the next, and yell at the nurses in between. They are overly dramatic with every single puny contraction, demand fresh bottled water, a refill on ice chips every twelve minutes, and constantly remind the nurses how incompetent they are. Now, your head is up your butt if you really think this encourages those nurses to give you the best care. No way, chicky. That nurse will roll her eyes and grimace at your every yoohoo. You are lucky if she actually cares enough to continue giving you any priority at all. At the very least, she's going to be curt, efficient but not doting, and try to get you out of there with as little contact as possible.

Yes, I know you are in dire pain and couldn't really give a rat's ass what that nurse thinks, but BITE YOUR TONGUE. Be pleasant or be quiet. And if you're not in labor, you have a much smaller basket of excuses.

Look, medical personnel in OB offices are used to complaints and overall pissed-off behavior toward the end of pregnancies, but that doesn't make them any more sympathetic or patient. And timid behavior doesn't help them meet your needs. Find that balance. Be nice and courteous, but assertive and secure. I promise, your care will be much more satisfactory if you communicate efficiently, effectively, and NICELY.

So. With that lecture out of the way, let's get on with the little joys you can expect on your visits (the ones where you are a sweet, adorable, kind little pregnant lady.)

Off to the Circus (Your First Visits): When you first discover you're pregnant, you'll want to immediately call and schedule an appointment. They may ask to see you right away to confirm your pregnancy, get an approximate due date, and do a yearly exam if you haven't had one recently. These visits are exciting in one sense, because you'll actually hear a professional say, "Congratulations!" but they are also quite similar to your yearly. You get weighed, pee in a cup, strip down, and have a breast and pelvic exam. Then comes the fun part. (What? You didn't think a hand up your hoochy-hoo was fun?) The doctor will do an internal exam and palpate your abdomen. Instead of saying, "Okay, everything looks good," he or she will tell you approximately how pregnant you are by the size of your uterus. Pretty cool!

Once all the nonsense is out of the way, your doctor will pull out that handy little date wheel to calculate your due date - and hound you for the first day of your last period. If you are like my friend Carey, you'll have a heck of a time coming up with that date. "Hmmm...um, maybe the last time it rained? Oh, wait, I know, it was the day Channel Four ran the story on the dog that water skis!" Needless to say, these mental landmarks are not exactly going to help. You'll need to give your doctor at least a smidgen of an idea when you started your last period, otherwise your due date will be a total guess based on your internal exam. Then you'll have to wait until your eight-week sonogram to get a good, solid date established. Aah! Torture!

Math Problems: I don't know about you, but I am perpetually confused on what to say when people ask, "How far along are you?" Do I give them weeks or months? Do I calculate from conception, or from the first day of my last period? On my first OB visit this time around, the doctor pronounced me four weeks pregnant based on my last period, examined me and said my uterus was at six-week size, then handed me a nifty pregnancy calendar which proclaimed me to be at the end of my fifth week. HUH?

The problem is that although pregnancy is defined by a 40-week period, it truly only lasts 38 weeks. As soon as you conceive, you automatically get two free weeks because your "pregnancy cycle" starts with the first day of your last period. Confusing? I agree, and having done this three times doesn't make it much less so. Suffice it to say that you can add two weeks to the gestational age of your embryo, and anyone familiar with pregnancy will know exactly where you're coming from. And if they don't have a clue, they're probably in the class of people like my dad and the dry cleaning clerk who truly don't care, so it doesn't matter.

As for whether to tell people months versus weeks, those in the pregnancy know will always go by weeks, and will in fact get confused if you say "five months" as opposed to "twenty weeks." Twenty weeks automatically lets us know that it's the half-way mark, whereas five months is more than half of nine months and doesn't make sense to those of us whose brains have been fried by pregnancy and motherhood.

Batter Up! (Sonograms): This is where it really gets good. The eight-week sonogram is the time when you first get to see the little bean in action. It's so dadgum sweet to see that tiny heartbeat and little webfeet and hands! I remember showing the sono picture of my first baby to my ten-year-old niece. I excitedly blurted, "The baby is about the size of a strawberry! Isn't that sweet?" So she took the picture and scrutinized - then handed it back to me and scoffed, "Your strawberry has a tail." Yes, okay, so the strawberry has a tail. It's still cute, thank you very much.

The cruddy thing about this sonogram is that it's not generally performed with an abdominal scanner. The baby is just too little to show up in enough detail. Instead, you will be delighted to know that you'll once again have to bare your bootie for a vaginal probe. If it sounds intimidating, well, it is. The thing is huge. It's basically a baseball bat. They stick this enormous "condom" on it, lube it up with jelly, and in it goes. Hello nasty!

The going in part isn't horrible. Uncomfortable, but not horrible. It's only when the doctor wrenches it around right and left that you'll start to mumble, "Ooh. Okay, pinch. Ow. Ouch!" Not a fun experience (unless you are into that sort of thing), but very necessary. The doctor will need to check your cervix as well as the heartbeat and make sure you don't have any stray babies hanging out on the sidelines.

In most uncomplicated pregnancies, you'll get another sono about halfway through, then one last sonogram at about 35 weeks. (And no vaginal probes! Woohoo!) By that time, body parts are fairly scrunched up in your little baby oven, so the kid probably won't be doing any amusing arm waves or twirls for you to coo over. However, the event itself is still an eye-opener. The entire point of the sono is to check for weight, fluid, or any red flags before delivery, but it's still just too fun to check out the facial features and try to decide who the baby looks like. With the blessed event being so close, we get insanely attached to our sonogram picture and show it to everyone from the bank teller to the mailman.

Appointment Jollies

For most of your pregnancy, you'll be required to check in with your practitioner only once a month. During these visits you'll get weighed, pee in a cup, and get your blood pressure taken. The staff will check the baby's heartbeat and ask some general questions about feet and hands swelling, bowel movements, or the like. (Yea, let's talk about crap!) Once the doctor comes in, you'll discuss any problems and concerns.

At about 16 weeks, they'll start measuring your uterus and possibly giving your abdomen a quick palpation. At around 25 weeks they will check your cervix to make sure it hasn't ruptured or dilated. And guess what this means! Yep! More hands up the Nuu-Nuu! Joy.

Your cervix will hopefully be nice and tight, but there are occasions when it's not. A nurse practitioner told me (in more ladylike terms than I am about to use) that she once stuck her glove up the wazoo and jumped out of her skin when a little hand grabbed her finger! (I seriously can't image how this happened, but I was too frightened to ask questions). Professionals wazoo lookers generally expect to feel a closed cervix. When they don't find it, they're only human and may startle a bit if Junior's trying to make an escape or giving a little fetus shout, "Hey wasup! And by the way, get your freaking hand outta here!" Do not panic if it happens to you. It's just a baby, not an alien.

By 30 weeks or so, you'll have to start going in for appointments every two weeks, and the last month you'll go every week. You'll basically get the same song and dance each visit, but they'll start checking your cervix each time once you hit the home stretch of about 35-36 weeks. Don't worry though. You'll get so used to all the poking and prodding that you'll hop your naked bum on the table, spread eagle, and think about as much of it as buying a loaf of bread.

These visits are all very routine and designed to catch any complications. They're still a source of fun and reassurance (aside from the weighing-in part and the hand up the hoochy-hoo), as you will get little updates every time you go in. Even if the information is just the baby's heart rate, you'll find comfort in knowing that your little one is packing on the weight right along with you and growing strong enough to wrestle a bull. If complications do arise, these visits give you the opportunity to communicate concerns and can provide peace of mind that all is progressing as well as possible.

Have You Felt the Baby Move? This is a question you will forever be asked, and it can be a bit perplexing. What does it feel like when the baby moves? If you are new to pregnancy, you may not be positive that the baby's movements are actually the baby's movements versus gas or some figment of your imagination. In the beginning, it's very difficult to tell because the movement can feel like anything from stomach "flutters" to pops like gas bubbles.

It's quite amusing actually – well, that is, if you're not throwing your guts up. The first time you feel something funny, you'll stop dead in your tracks and think, "Was that it?" You'll grab anyone standing nearby, forcing them to feel your belly and give a second opinion. If you're really skinny you can actually lie flat on your back and see your belly move. This can be strange, exciting, and creepy all at the same time.

Feeling a baby move is literally like getting used to a tadpole swimming around in your stomach. At first, there's tiny fin flips. Then the little fish starts making bubbles. Before you know it, the growing critter has morphed into a frog and hops all over your belly, spinning, kicking, twirling, and grooving. By the end of the second trimester, it feels like there's an octopus in there — eight arms swirling and slithering around. And hitting the third trimester is just something you'll have to experience to believe. Bones are stronger, the kid is squished, and you will definitely be convinced that not only is there a real, live baby in there, but he's surely got a girlfriend. With all the karate kicks and belly punches, you'll be hard pressed to imagine that only four limbs can make all that fuss.

So when your doctor asks, "Have you felt the baby move?" go ahead and describe your symptoms, even if you aren't sure. As your pregnancy progresses, they'll want to know if the movement increases, decreases, or stays the same. Sometimes you may even be required to do a "kick count" where you count the number of kicks within a certain time frame, usually ten minutes. You record it on a little sheet and dutifully bring it to your visits for the doctor to assess.

The only time you should be concerned is if you've noticed a marked decrease in the movement. Keep in mind that if you've been busy running around and haven't noticed one way or the other, that doesn't count. Unless the kid is starving and banging the walls for food, you'll probably be distracted enough that you won't notice much movement. It's only when you've settled down and you're really paying attention. Ask your doctor for specifics on when to call, because it varies throughout your pregnancy, but (very) generally you are looking for movement everyday in the second trimester and several times an hour by the third.

Now that I've scared you silly, please remember that I am *not* a doctor. My advice is only girlfriend to girlfriend. _Always_ consult your doctor when you have any concerns. That said, I must tell you that I myself have noticed a bit of decreased movement lately, but I've also used common sense in not freaking out. Deciding that my sugar intake has been off the charts and needs to slow down, I've increased my protein and decreased my crap-intake by more than half. And guess what? Baby has calmed down. Not because something is wrong, but because I'm not putting my poor child into sugar-spasms by eating candy bars, cake, cookies, and ice cream three times a day. I've been complaining for quite a while that this kid is crazy-busy in there, and it's really no wonder with how addicted I was to sugar.

That Nasty Glucose Test: Since we're on the topic of sugar, we may as well discuss that horrible test for gestational diabetes. Somewhere in the middle of your second trimester, your practitioner will give you a huge bottle of something that looks like orange soda. Your instructions are to drink a prescribed amount within five minutes, don't eat anything after, and race to the doctor's office to have your blood drawn exactly one hour after the last nasty sip.

Doesn't sound so dreadful? Well. Hmph. Honey, this drink is sickening. Not that it's loaded with ground-up worms or liquefied lettuce, but being chock full of glucose, the sweetness makes it nauseating. However, I do have to admit that it's not as bad as it used to be. During my last two pregnancies, I had to fast before drinking the gnarly excuse for orange soda. Talk about making you want to puke and faint – whew! This time around, I could eat before drinking it, and thank God for small favors.

I actually asked, pleaded, then got downright snooty in my attempts to get out of this test. But my doctor was stone. No can do. My teeny-tiny, black-belt, all muscle, ninety-five-pound doctor got very assertive and absolutely insisted I be a good patient and do as I'm told. Why? Because having gestational diabetes can mean serious diet changes to deliver a healthy baby. Those women delivering premature eleven-pound babies? Yep. That's the least of what you're looking at if you don't know you're glucose intolerant. This test is really an easy way to determine if there's a very treatable condition going on. So be brave. Suck it up, suck it down, and get it over with. (And by the way, no joke on the black-belt doctor. She even showed up one time with a black eye. Seeing my horrified expression, she smiled and matter-of-factly reported, "You gotta learn to block!" referring to a recent class. Holy moly gazoly!)

Braxton-Hicks: Here's another possible discomfort throughout your pregnancy, and a source of the endless question, "Have you had any contractions?" With first pregnancies, it's a real pickle of a query. Never having had to use your uterus before, knowing what a contraction feels like is quite impossible. And some women never even get a twinge until the big moment arrives. My friend Lorraine said she went about her merry way with both of her pregnancies, and as soon as that belly started tightening up, she knew "it was time."

On the other side of the equation, I get contractions all the time — irritates the snot out of me. They come on when I move suddenly, rest, exercise, eat, drive, type, or sneeze. There are consistently 20-25 per day, and they're worse and rather painful at night if I'm exceptionally worn out. (And please. What's "exceptional"? I'm always worn out.)

What do they feel like? Well, if you can imagine a huge ball in your belly, try to picture the ball getting tight, firm, and slightly smaller. Now think about the ball being attached to, and tugging on, all of your stomach muscles. It will also pull your back muscles forward and put enough pressure on your lungs to make it slightly difficult to breathe. When you have a Braxton-Hicks contraction, your belly will get very hard and you may have to stop moving and center yourself.

Having always read that these contractions are not painful, I'd like to take some time and get on my box. Maybe they aren't terribly *painful*, but they are definitely high up on the scale of *uncomfortable*. During one of these contractions, I can still walk (*ve-ry* slowly), breathe, and carry on a limited conversation, but I usually don't. I'm too busy grabbing anything or anyone in range, making Mr. Grimace-face, and yoga breathing my way through it. If this is your first pregnancy, Braxton-Hicks contractions really shouldn't be this bad. It's only when you've cranked out a couple of kids and your uterus is officially old and cranky that they get irritating and edge toward "painful."

They are so strong and frequent for me, in fact, that toward the end of my pregnancies, people get extremely nervous. My friend Amy will always give me bug-eyed squeaks, "Okay, how am I supposed to know if this is the real deal or not?!" The pat answer is that when I start to cry, it's the real deal. She can then feel free to haul my hippo-butt to the nearest hospital.

Where's Your Head, Man? (Presentation of the Baby): Your doctor will be checking for the presentation of the baby throughout your pregnancy. They're looking for a head-down position. With many first pregnancies, the baby is head down very early on, so it's not an issue. However, for a small percentage of women, the baby will be breech (head up). This causes a problem in that you don't want to try and force out a baby that's butt or feet first. You would think that if they can come out head first, they should be able to come out the opposite way and do fine too. Sometimes that's possible, but many doctors in this age of malpractice suits aren't going to risk it, and I can't say as I blame them. If, for any reason, the baby's head should get stuck in your pelvis with the rest of the body out, well, this is just all around *bad* news. You would do well to avoid the possibility at all costs.

I've known a couple of women now whose first babies didn't turn head down until two to four weeks before delivery. That's cutting it pretty close, but close counts in this case. Some doctors will get antsy and want to put you through a rather involved and "uncomfortable" (that term again) procedure called External Cephalic Version (ECV). The goal of an ECV is to turn the baby if it doesn't turn on its own by 36 weeks or so. This procedure calls for externally maneuvering the baby in your uterus. There is some risk involved since the baby's heart rate can drop. Because of this, some doctors will want to attempt this procedure in an operating room with an anesthesiologist standing by in case they deem an emergency C-section is necessary.

Unless your hubby happens to be an OB and turns the baby himself as you lie comfortably on your own bed (yes, I know someone who has done this!), an ECV will go somewhat along these lines: You get hooked up to an I.V., given medication to relax your uterus, and the doctor checks the baby's position through a sonogram. They then start pushing, prodding, and squeezing away, trying to get the kid to turn. This can be a no-big-deal-relax-and-enjoy-the-ride kind of thing or a puke potential for squeamish souls.

Having my own stinker of a breech baby, my doctor tried to prepare me for an ECV in case the baby didn't turn. Anxiety high, I consulted anyone and everyone on how I could get this kid to flop and avoid the drama. When my doctor first told me, "You need to figure out a way to get this kid to turn," my first thought was, "What the heck do you want me to do? Stand on my head?" "Yes," according to my Poker Mommy Carey. She said to get in a pool, do a handstand, and stay there for as long as I could. Amy quickly piped in that she'd pay me twenty bucks if I'd actually do it and she could witness. I mean...what? What the hell kind of help is this?

Other advice included eating a peanut butter and jelly sandwich (no, I'm not kidding), or squatting like a baseball catcher while watching T.V. The sandwich theory was given in all seriousness, as the woman who suggested it was thoroughly convinced those two pieces of bread actually turned her kid at 36 weeks. She flopped on the couch, ate the sandwich, and cried out in panic as her belly promptly contorted and twisted in sci-fi movie fashion. And the squatting advice was given to "open up" the pelvic region and encourage Jr. to head towards the door.

Ok, really. So what is a normal, rational, pregnant woman to do with all this nonsense advice? Try it, of course. I was thoroughly desperate so I gave two out of three a whirl. (Sorry Carey, but I'll skip standing on my head, thank you very much. I can't even bend over to pick up a shoe without every pint of blood in my body rushing to my head. A handstand would murder my overworked nasal passages.)

Anyway, I ended up having the ECV. (What? You're surprised?) It was definitely a big deal – four hours at the hospital as they prepped me, monitored the baby, performed the procedure, and monitored the baby some more. Only when they were thoroughly convinced I wasn't going to go into labor and the kid wasn't flopping back to the original position, they let me go home. And you know what? It worked. The general success rate is moderate, and it IS very uncomfortable (okay, it hurts), but the end result of being able to deliver vaginally makes it worth the effort and discomfort.

The Art of Peeing in a Cup

Think me a lunatic all you want, but I promise, as your belly inflates, peeing in a cup becomes an Olympic challenge. First of all, the swollen woo-woo makes aim a thing of the past. Urine just sort of shoots all over the place, drenching you, your hand, and the cup you're peeing in. Then, as your stomach starts to resemble the tip of a torpedo, reaching underneath your belly to the target area becomes a feat worthy of Stretch-Man himself. You can forget attempting to see anything going on down there or shooting for a visual approximation of hitting that cup. It's a waste of time and neck strain.

As a veteran of cup-peeing, let me clue you in and make your life much less frustrating. Get the cup in the general vicinity and press it up on your peanut like you're trying to suction the darn thing to your body. That's the only way to catch the wayward pee and avoid soaking your hand. When you get enough in the specimen cup, wipe down the rim and outside with a paper towel to ensure you don't gross out the nurses. I'm sure they see much worse throughout the day, but don't give them a reason to be in a pissy mood when they take your weight and blood pressure.

Hate You, Hate You, Skinny Witch!

Here we go again with the weight business. We've covered the basics of how much to gain and when, so we'll skip that depressing part and get on to reality — when you're gaining too much. You may actually be right on target with putting on the pounds, but you'll still *feel* like it's too much. This is especially true for women who start out very thin or who maintain a very steady and relatively healthy weight when not pregnant. Putting on extra pounds is just so darned uncomfortable and worrisome that it can very well ruin your day each time you have to step on that blasted scale.

Listen up, girlfriend! Don't let weight gain get to you. Get over yourself. And hey, I know how hard it is when you are literally surrounded by pictures of skinny be-otches. The media is dead set on convincing women how they "should" look and pointing out all of our inadequacies in order to sell us the latest and greatest cellulite cream, gym memberships, and diet pills. Pay attention and hear me well all ye gestating women: *It's all a scam!* You know as well as I do that most normal people don't look like those anorexic chics on magazine covers, and we don't go around sporting five hundred dollar designer shoes and Prada bags. It's just not reality. Sure, some people really do indulge and live it up. Kuddos and more power to 'em. Just don't go thinking you have to measure up, because you don't.

The last time I was in the doctor's office, I picked up one of those generic pregnancy magazines and nearly had a stroke just staring at the cover. Here was this pregnant professional model and athlete –all six feet, five inches of her– beautifully tan, perfect skin and hair, showing off this teeny tiny bump by sporting a bikini that I wouldn't be caught dead in on the best non-pregnant day of my life. Turns out, this teeny tiny bump was about to pop as she was almost due to give birth when she shot that cover. I could have died. Floop! Saint Peter, here I come. Was that really and truly what I was supposed to look like? My world went to hell in a hand basket right there in that office. I literally had to talk myself out of weeping over some stupid cover shot.

Here's the deal, ladies. My reaction to that picture was the entire point of putting that beautiful woman on the cover. I anxiously stared, worried that I wasn't worthy of being pregnant, and considered buying every single freaking product that magazine had to sell in order to get myself looking as spiffy as that model. I was positively itching to read the article to find out how she maintained her figure and where she got that fabulous suit – the works. *That's* what sells the magazine, and the people writing those articles and shooting those pictures know it damn well. It DOES NOT MEAN that the rest of us are supposed to look like that cover model. It is fine and dandy to pick up the magazine, learn all you can about the birthing experiences of others, and get a feel for the products and medical care available for you and your baby. Just don't buy into the notion that we need to be as attractive as that (dadgum) model.

Your pregnant body is beautiful. May I repeat myself? *Your pregnant body is beautiful.* DO NOT let some image of the "perfect" gestating vessel sway you into thinking differently. You are assisting Nature in a miracle here, and there is nothing more beautiful on this Earth. Let me remind you that although models are all toothpicks and gorgeous genetic mutants, they also have the advantage of photo re-imaging.

Never forget that the lovely ladies on magazine covers are touched up so much that editors might as well digitally create the entire photo and save themselves the hassle of forking over the big bucks to Ms. Skinny Pants. Butts can be firmed, dark circles removed, hair color and outfits changed, and models stretched to look taller and thinner. Computer wizards can even deftly mix and match heads with bodies.

The truth of the matter is that pictures do not denote reality. There's no more truth in photos, girly! My best friend touches up her own family photos lickety-split. She just gets on her computer, pulls up the image, and changes whatever she wants. She's made her lips colorful, fixed a gimp eye, even given herself longer bangs. So the next time you see some stunning picture in a magazine or on T.V., assume it's been so edited that it hardly resembles the actual person. I guarantee if you were to hunt this chic down and force her to take off all her make-up and sewn-on clothes, she'd look pretty darn close to a normal person. That means *you*, dear!

Yes, being hugely pregnant can be depressing. I concede you may very well feel like a milking cow and detest putting on clothes each morning for fear of busting seams. But the reality is that you are making a baby. Feel as miserable as you like. Brood, growl, snap, and cry over every pound you gain. It's not going to help. Your body is going to morph into someone you don't know, and that's all there is to it.

Now, I'm certainly not saying you should throw in the towel and bury yourself in mayo-slathered BLT's. Don't get too depressed to care, because it certainly won't do much to boost the ol' self esteem. Take care of your body and baby, but don't beat yourself up if you aren't staying within some ideal image. Eat right, exercise, keep your hair and make-up nice, wear clothes that make you feel good, and embrace your pregnant self. Remember, you are the one who is most critical of yourself. Other people don't see the flaws you do, so give it up and stop worrying. As much as I bitch and complain, it's all in fun. I promise, you look a lot better than you think.

Chapter Seven: Last Trimester Love Fest

Oooooh, mercy. This last mile stretch is...long. I'm tired. And cranky. So let's get this going and get this over with because I. Am. Done.

Pediatricians

Finding a pediatrician should be high on your last trimester to-do list. However, don't fret if it slips your mind. The hospital will supply one after birth if you don't have one picked out.

How to Choose & When to Switch: Get some recommendations and interview a few good ones. You'd be surprised how you can make an I-don't-like-you assessment in 30 seconds flat. Better not to be stuck with a dud when baby's sick and you're desperate for help. My friend Melanie had a doc who put her 6-month-old son on antibiotics for a month for a stubborn lump on his bum. Dr. Fright painfully squeezed the goo out of it and gave Melanie sermons about antibiotic-resistant staph, scaring her to death. But guess what? No results except needless pain and drugs. Melanie finally switched pediatricians. The next doc took one look and said her son needed out-patient surgery for an anal fissure. Problem solved.

You need to be proactive about your baby's health. Pediatricians are generalists who only know/tell you so much. For example, my friend Kristi will pounce on anyone in lecture distance, yammering about breastfed babies being vitamin D deficient. She claims massive studies are touting the benefits of vitamin D. While it's easy to supplement, you have to actually know about it first. And of course, she's a bit peeved that her doctors never mentioned it. Her son ended up with Type 1 diabetes. She doesn't assert that vitamin D deficiency contributed to this, because nobody knows. But she'll get on a box about studies where therapeutic doses of vitamin D reduced Type 1 diabetes rates by 80%. If she'd known, she would've supplemented, and she still feels guilty. Just keep in mind that doctors are there to answer your pressing questions, not fill you in on every healthcare detail and put you on a personalized plan for optimum health. That's our job, Mommies!

Gobbledy-Gook (A Host of Pleasures)

Speak English! In addition to being cranky and just a wee bit sensitive, we also won't make much sense. Purple shoe on big fairy lights. (Uh huh.) Being preoccupied with the upcoming miracle is enough to crowd all other nonsense out of our brain. The expressive result is often a sort of pregnant gibberish.

The only solution to this mental block (which, sorry to tell you, doesn't get much better with initiation to Motherhood) is to accept that you are not your normal self, tell all others around you to ignore your ranting, and get as much sleep as you can. Don't overload yourself with errands, setting up the nursery, and writing thank-you cards. When people offer to help, put them to work! They'll actually be very happy to *do* something other than sit around, twiddling their thumbs, waiting for you to pop. You might also stop whining about how much you need to do if you can order people around to do it for you. They'll love it; any kind of busy activity is better than hanging around listening to us make no sense whatsoever.

Back Pain: Oooh, the constant aching, pinching, and disabling soreness! Why? Why us? My own relief is rare, and it doesn't matter what I do. By the time it gets dark outside, I'm practically crying in my desperation for the pain to go away. Sleep helps. Exercise too. I do "assisted squats" to strengthen my back and legs. It's best to have a trainer or professional at your gym show you the correct way to do it, but I'll explain it just to give you a mental picture. Get one of those huge exercise balls, place it about chest level on a wall, then turn around and lean your back up against it. Position it low so that when you squat, the ball won't roll up to your head, pop right out from under your weight, and flop you to the ground. Once the ball is in place, squat down into a sitting position, then slowly stand back up. The ball will roll with you and make the whole process bearable. This exercise is easy and builds your strength a bit. I can do several sets of twenty-five before pooping out. I rest in between sets (sitting on the ball, of course) and quit when I'm tired. Ask your doctor if this exercise would be good for you and your particular aches and pains.

Sleep: Depending on how much your appendages stick out and where, sleep can be an elusive thing. Being all-over kind of big is not fun since the groaning mattress reminds you every time you lay down. Having a missile poking out from your midriff is no picnic either, considering the awesome task of turning from side to side. And, you cannot lie on your back lest you risk crushing yourself to death; the pressure is too much for your lungs and spine and decreases good blood flow to the baby.

So side-lying it is, a rather uncomfortable proposition. We've talked about positioning pillows and making the most of your discomfort, but Lord have mercy. The third trimester problem is when you tire of resting on one side and need to flop over to the other. This entails wrenching your arm under the offending side of your belly and literally slinging it over to the other side. You must simultaneously shift hips and cheeks and use your feet to help launch the scud. The volcanic commotion is quite a sight, but don't you dare laugh, or I will be forced to fart on you. Once I can make it off this bed.

Nesting: Okay, forget aching back, swollen feet, and the severe need for a bikini wax. Dadgum if this gardening isn't getting done TODAY. Dig that dirt! Plant those flowers! Mow that grass! And when that's done, it's on to organizing: closets, drawers, cubbies, and furniture. Speaking of, what IS it with our intense need to move furniture?? I don't know why – but that bed really, really does need to move to the other side of the room. As in, now. And the couch – it's just gotta go this way, not that. It sounds so illogical, but I swear if it doesn't get done right this minute, you will rue the day, mister!

You know, perhaps this is Mother Nature's way of getting us off our cans. We can assert the activity is only to get us dilating, but the truth is, it's just one of those *things*. We can't help it. Our hubbies, in the valiant attempt to look after their gestating vessels, will bellow orders to "stop that or else!" But gawl-ly! I can't stop! Can you? A nervous personality to begin with, if you tell me I can't do something that I'm positive needs to be done – hells bells.

So what do we do? Order people around, that's what! Grab those towel-twisting, nervous-nelly, family members hovering about and set them to it. Make them move stuff all day long. At the very least it will be entertaining and keep our mind off our need to ... Wait. I need to go eat.

I'll Never Make it!

You will either refuse to believe or have forgotten entirely the incredible stretching power of your uterus. Even with baby number two and three, you'll lament, *"I'll never make it!"* with the exact same sincerity each time. Obviously, I'm on your side with this one. I for one am just positive that my belly really does get bigger with each pregnancy. Not believing that it can actually *do* that makes each gestating process all the more alarming.

I know for a fact that I am quite beyond comprehension, because Mothers-To-Be get quite frightened at the sight of my ripe middle. Even those who've had several kids get extremely nervous seeing me waddle around, especially now. All day, every day, I get the "Oh honey, you look miserable" and "Oh my gosh, are you going to make it?" comments. I'm quite sick of it. Not only do I loathe struggling to do the most basic tasks like getting in and out of my car, but I have to contend with everyone around me acting extremely grateful they aren't in my shoes. And some jackasses think it's simply hilarious to joke about you being a watermelon. (Yeah, that's just too funny.) For the most part, they are kind, and it's very nice of people to show concern for my condition, but it gets to be a constant reminder of how much it stinks to get through each day.

My advice to you? Suck up all the positive attention you can get, and ignore the people who act like you're a walking time bomb. Women who've been there will make sweet and empathetic comments. Eat that up like candy. Just pay no heed to the idiots who huff and gasp at the sight of you. Although you can't really blame them for the astonished reaction, they still don't have enough couth to keep it to themselves. They are therefore not in the category of pregnant-friendly people. Surround yourself with those lovely ladies who've been there and done that, and bask in their loving and encouraging words. Your race is almost over and you will soon be among the sympathizers. Isn't that a wonderful thought?

Sex? Are you kidding!?

After taking a very unscientific poll, the results are in. Pregnancy hormones seem to throw sex into two categories: Can't Get Enough, or Go Away. Some of you gals may have closed the deli and told hubby to take his business elsewhere for a while. Quite rational, given our diving self esteem, rolly-polly body, and just plain "keep that thing away from me" mind set. But the rest of you are on an orgasm jag, making your husband wonder what happened to his wife. Not that he's complaining, because a whole new sex partner is fantasy town, but working him to death and loving every minute is just plain weird. This is the double-orgasm, climax-in-your-sleep, think-about-it-all-the-time kind of hormones. You're liable to have a herky-jerky just brushing your teeth! You'll find yourself doing daily crazies like getting on the treadmill butt naked, or doing the dishes in a thong in hopes of enticing your man yet one more time.

But now you're in the third trimester. Newsflash! Third trimester sex has significant difficulties, especially that last month. Here's the thing. You've got two choices: Off-To-The-Side or Brave-The-Fanny.

Off-To-The-Side: This seems logical. You used to be able to copulate just fine. You'd think if hubby could just move around the belly and flop his top half to one side or the other, he'd still be able to thread the needle, no problem. Well, okay, maybe a couple of problems. First off, God love him, here's to hoping your husband doesn't have a gut. And

111

even if he doesn't, you could still end up flapping bellies like fish. Slap, slap, slap. Ugh.

Second, this method is rather like jamming a frozen hotdog sideways in a bun – the logistics are quite baffling. Not much fun having a sausage ram-rod the walls of your hoochy-hoo. And I know this is horribly graphic, but what I am supposed to do?! Decency was thrown out the window just as soon as the topic was introduced. How else do you talk about this stuff? (I'll ask my mom. Ho ho! You know, I love a good, supportive mom, but Lord in heaven, I hope her royal Catholic-ness never reads one word of this book. I'll be damned for sure. She'll say rosaries for me daily.)

Brave-The-Fanny: This method is probably easier. Sure, hubby still has to navigate our enormous behinds, but chances are good that it's smaller surface space than the front. Getting the arrow on the bullseye shouldn't be too hard either. It's so freaking big that you'd have to be clueless as to what the target even looks like before you could possibly miss *that*.

So lay on your side, get a pillow between your knees, and make hubby work around your comfort. He can twist and contort his non-pregnant skinny butt much better than you, so leave any "figuring out how to get it done" to him. Without five huge mirrors, you can't possibly know what's going on back there, anyway, and heaven knows it's probably not pretty. So get as comfy as possible and let him have at it. I'd advise YOU not get too into it, though, as orgasms tighten up your uterus like a vise. If you're trying to get this show on the road and coming along healthy as a horse, that's different. Have fun and contract away. Otherwise, lay your head on that pillow and take a snooze - if you don't mind the boat rocking.

Coconut in the Crotch: The Baby Drops

Can anyone say, "coconut between your legs?" That is exactly what it feels like; a coconut right where a tampon should be. And no, it's not literally where a tampon takes residence, otherwise the kid would be falling out, but this is as close as it gets. And hello waddles-ville! Trying to navigate your legs without crushing your baby's head is a trick. This doesn't seem humanly possible, but you basically walk around in a quarter squat, dragging and looping each leg forward in the pathetic attempt to put one foot in front of the other. Quite miserable, HOWEVER, there is an awesome silver lining. We can breathe, baby! Aaaah, suck in that sweet air, because Jr. has now abandoned his lung-crushing post. Woopie! So breathe deep and...don't walk. Yeah. You'll be good. Make lovie-dovie with the couch and take it easy.

Chapter Eight: Get This Show on the Road

Never having been in labor before, it can be quite a riddle as to when the big moment has come. Do you go to the hospital or not? Should you call the doctor instead? When should hubby jump in his car and race home from work? Is it okay to call your mother in the middle of the night with the first twang of a real contraction?

If it makes you feel any better, these questions forever loom in the mind of the "due" lady. It doesn't matter if it's baby number one or baby number four. Each pregnancy is different and therefore unpredictable. And we're all just positive that this has to end soon or we'll collapse under the elephant weight and emotional strain. The following are some indications that your beautiful day has truly come and you are on your way to Mommy-dom.

Contractions (The Real Deal): Technically speaking, real contractions, as opposed to the falsy Braxton-Hicks, are defined by whether or not they get you dilating. Real contractions dilate the cervix, fake ones don't. Is it easy to tell the difference? That depends. If you haven't had any Braxton-Hicks to compare the real ones to, and you have no idea what a contraction feels like to begin with, well, no, it's not that easy. Every woman is different, too. Some have a high pain threshold (or a very happy uterus) and can be dilating away while thinking, "Huh. I'm a tad bit uncomfortable today!" Others can have contractions making us curse all the way to the hospital and keeping us yelling profanities for the next ten hours, as our cervix takes its sweet time opening up the gate so the royal subject can finally make an appearance.

Real dilation-worthy contractions are generally always painful. Yes, you will find the occasional yogini-ultra-centered-totally-in-tune-with-her-body chic that will claim contractions don't have to hurt, that they can simply be a "feeling" or "sensation" your body goes through. To that I say, "Good for you. Now go and take your happy, painless cheer for a walk around the block, please."

Look, I'm all for natural ways to go about this birthing business – a firm believer in the brain's ability to heal and control pain. But personally, it's not happening with me. Take your party outside because no one is talking me out of a nice epidural cocktail just because we should be more "one" with our body. Forget that crap. Quick and painless is my motto. Agree or not, and go for it if you are strong, motivated, and centered enough to try natural methods of pain control. I'll be your biggest cheerleader and personal advocate. Just don't be that chic who bravely refuses pain meds for everything including a root canal, yet starts the nails-on-a-chalkboard screaming business when the rest of us are in the next labor room trying to peacefully reach our ten centimeters. Believe me, there'll always be *someone* in the next room screeching in pain while you're calmly trying to labor. It's freaking scary to the rest of us, girlfriend!

Back to contractions. Those that get you good and dilated are going to feel intense. Exactly how intense and where you'll have the pain, you won't know until you're there. They can range from knife-jabbing, son-of-a-bitch sensations anywhere on your belly or crotch, to massive leg aches and/or total "back labor" where you are positive your back is simply going to break in half. Whatever the "sensation" (can I laugh now?), your belly will get hard as a rock and you won't be able to talk (although shouting is feasible), move, or listen to anyone else jabber in your ear. One woman I knew insisted her husband count during contractions, but got so fed up with the sound of his voice that she hissed, "Stop that counting!" Two contractions later, he's sulking in the corner of the room and she roars, "You're supposed to be counting!"

Contractions that dilate are usually painful. Call it what you wish, but I don't think those typical-book-cutesy terms come close to describing Mother Nature hard at work. Your cervix must dilate to ten times the normal size and your baby must squeeze out of body parts that aren't exactly made of elastic. (By the way, that old phrase "your body will open up like a flower" is a bunch of horse crap. Yeah, it opens up like a flower all right – an angry, inflamed, ripped-open pissed-off flower.)

Basically, real contractions hurt like hell, and you'll know when it's upon you.

Now that I've terrified you, relax. You'll get through it. Everyone does. I even have a friend who is so petrified of receiving drugs or an epidural that she voluntarily goes through the pain of childbirth and nary says a word about it. She knows it will hurt like a big dog but clenches her teeth and plows through because she feels the alternatives are worse. Now that is grit! You go girl.

The thing that is most "painful" about contractions is not the contractions themselves, but the fear that goes along with it. With your first kid, you have no idea what to expect and it's downright scary. Fear of the unknown is the biggest obstacle to overcome. The pain is bad, but we are women and we can take it. It's the lead up to the big event that scares the bejeebies out of us. I'm not much into childbirth classes, but I do know that many of them address this and try to calm your fears. When that is accomplished, you've come a long way in dealing with the pain.

Once you've figured out that these are the real deal, use your doctor's recommendations on when to hit the hospital or birthing center. Many use a 411 rule: the old standby of contractions that are 4 minutes apart, lasting one minute each, for one hour. Use your judgment on these, though, because for most women I've talked to, contractions are all over the place. And by the time they're that frequent, little miss pansy here will want that epidural nice and flowing.

Dilation and Effacement: During that last month, you will most likely have to hit the doctor's office every week so they can check your cervix – is the old girl getting ripe, or what? Each and every time you waddle your gigantic self in there, you think, oh ye god of dilating cervixes, please let it be - and get this kid out! And those cheerful doctors will smile and say, "Okay, you're about 25% effaced!" Or, with subsequent pregnancies, you usually dilate first, so they'll pipe up in that annoyingly chipper voice, "Two centimeters! Not long now!" Ooooh, glory be and halleluiah! It's coming! It's almost over!

Hold on there, honey bunches. Exasperating news. Doctors and nurses must throw us a bone every once in a while, otherwise we'd beat them with a stick to *do something* and get this thing going. This is their "do something." It's the doctor's lollipop to impatient mothers-to-be. I'm just positive they've all conspired and made up this whole early dilation/effacement business just to give us anxious women something to do. Why am I so suspicious? Because I've been walking around three centimeters dilated and almost fully effaced for what seems like two weeks now, and this baby isn't anywhere near coming out. With all the contractions I'm having, everyone around me is on pins and needles thinking the pig's going to pop right in front of them. But *nooo*. Baby's staying put.

I've tried everything. I walk (okay, drag my legs around) to stimulate labor. I demand my gracious husband navigate my belly and deposit his cervix-softening sperm every other day (poor guy). I even ask for "rough" exams. During a rough exam, or "stripping the membranes," the doctor will try and stimulate your cervix by rubbing it with a little more gusto when checking for dilation. Does it work? Heck no. At least not in my case. All it does is irritate my already-angry uterus. I'll have piddly, do-nothing, painful contractions and feel like I've got the flu for about twelve hours. Then zippo. Nada. Next visit, no change. Not worth it in my opinion.

On the optimistic side (which I'll try to be, despite my misery, for your sake) this can actually sometimes be a great indicator of labor. Go ahead and think positive. Call your family, be happy, and send good vibes down the belly. Maybe you can *will* that kid out. Start preparing, if for no other reason than to give you something to do.

Either way, when you begin to dilate, you'll want to start changing your habits and eating lighter. During the last few weeks of pregnancy you'll get sick eating the same amount of food as you have for the past six months. Aside from the fact that there's simply no more room in your stomach, your body seems to know it's time to slow down and will pass the memo on to you. Also, if it's truly crunch time, ease up on the heavy foods so you won't die of heartburn - or embarrassment - as you yak it up on the delivery bed.

Train to Grossville (Plug Passing & Other Joys)

Oh, joy of joys! Now, if this wasn't fun, I can't tell you what is!! And thank you VERY much, all you advice-giver doctors and authors, for skimming over this abomination. You put lipstick on this pig for me one more time, and I WILL start punching.

What's the problem, you ask? Oh, I'll tell you the problem. So I'm in the bathroom, not a festive event to begin with. I go to wipe my already slimy banana, and SWEET HOLY MOSES AND GREAT BALLS OF FIRE! This humongo glob of just... blood-streaked YUCK...attaches its nastiness to my tissue wad and just keeps coming and coming as I yank and wipe, yank and wipe. I had to grab the wall to keep from fainting. You know, I thought I had seen slime and goo. This is my third time around, and whether you want to hear it or not, my body puts it out like an alien with a sinus infection. But this! This was just too much.

Never having experienced this happiness before, thank heavens I at least had some inkling of what it was. Otherwise my head was hitting that porcelain. My husband would have found me two hours later, pants down around my ankles, looking like a ghoul from Ghostbusters sneezed on me. I was so upset that I nearly pinned my doctor to the wall on my next visit. "You better tell me I'm in labor because I passed my plug and nearly fainted and you didn't tell me it would be that gross and 'bloody show' is bloody right, and get your hand up there and check!!" She just smiled sheepishly, "Oh, you didn't like that part, huh?" No SHIT, Sherlock! Groooooosss!

Flu-Like Symptoms: Poo-poo time! Generally miserable, achy, crampy, and seriously tired, feeling more-down-in-the-dumps than usual can mean that happy day is coming soon. Not that you care, because, well, you're feeling so crappy. Sometimes you can have indigestion, nausea, or vomiting as well. As long as you don't have a fever, don't panic. Just stay on the couch or bed, and lug yourself up only long enough to hit the toilet to yak or blow those bowels as needed. I am always more than happy to have near-diarrhea toward the end. My fear of disgusting my husband out of our master bathroom is nothing compared to pooping on the doctor during delivery. I say, bring it on and get that unhappy colon cleared out!

Poopin' on the Doc: I think this topic is a bit less taboo than it used to be, but seriously, how many women have you met that casually go, "Oh yeah. Happened to me."? Volunteering your everyone-saw-me-poop horror story is still not the norm. And those standard pregnancy books stick in one measly, technical paragraph on how your muscles relax and the baby squishes out any leftover bowel...whatever. Girlfriend, it's pretty likely you'll push out a log on your doctor, and that's that. Bare, naked, awful truth. You don't mean to, but honey, you have no earthly idea it's even happening, so don't sweat it.

Your entire pelvic floor will be hurting so intensely that you really won't care what's coming out of your body, nor will you be aware. That is, of course, unless you get an epidural. Then you'll be feeling good enough to have a mild concern about how you look spread eagle and squirting unmentionables. Not a pleasant thought, I know, but you've got to make room for that baby somewhere. Holding your bowel contents is not a priority at this time!

Don't wait until you're pushing, but if you feel so inclined, think ahead. For my last two pregnancies, I've made clearing that butt a top priority, and have no intention of changing that now. I always schedule inductions, though, as I am positive my babies will never come out unless they are forced (and by golly, I want them OUT). I load up on the prune juice the night before. With the best luck in the world, my bowels have happily expelled right before heading to the hospital each time so far. Hopefully the same will happen this go round.

We always wait to find out the sex of the baby until they pop out, so of course my first question is, "What is it?!" but the second frantic question is, "Did I poop?!" Everyone is so goo-goo eyed over the baby that they could care less about hurting my feelings, so I figure it's a good time to ask. So far the answer has been "No, you were fine" each time, but who can believe? I can see my husband overlooking it since he's totally cool with blood and gore. And my doctors - well, not that they're liar-liar-pants-on-fire, but they're so busy pulling and sewing that I doubt they even hear my mewing question. They probably just mumble whatever they think is appropriate enough to shut me up.

I keep telling you to relax about it, but I'm the world's biggest hypocrite. Even this time around, the thought of it gives me the willies of dread, so I'm downing the prune juice and keeping that enema handy. If prune juice doesn't work and you chicken-out on the enema, you can always ask the nurse for one once you get to the hospital. I'm sure they'll love you to pieces after that. But if you can't bring yourself to navigate the butt cheeks and stick something up your own keister, whadiya gonna do?

Breaking Water: So I carry around a towel. Not that the Smith water bag has ever broken on its own, I just still have this intense fear of some stranger having to clean up my former innards. Everywhere I go, the towel goes too; car, bed, store, couch. When sitting, it goes under my butt, and when standing, next to my purse. My husband is more embarrassed about the towel than the thought of me squirting bodily fluids on his family members, but that's his problem.

Water will usually break when you're standing and the baby's head is pressing down on a little pouch of fluid caught in between his head and your cervix. When you're lying down, gravity isn't ram-rodding his head into your cervical door like Black Friday shoppers. Unless you've got some serious contractions or this-is-it-you're-gonna-need-to-push-soon, the probability of gushing while horizontal is low. Nonetheless, I sleep on a towel!

If water does break, it can be a trickle or a gush. I'm sure you know all about this already, so I won't go into huge detail, but it shouldn't be a torrent. If you have on clothes, it should just get them wet, not spill to the ground like you've been dumped with a bucket. My Poker Mommy Carey says her water loves to break in the shower. Plooosh! How lucky is that?! But no matter how it comes out, if it's green, get your ass to the hospital.

Speaking of the hospital, if it hasn't broken by then and your doctor wants to move things along, he/she can stick a little hook in there and do it manually. It scares me to death every time. Lord knows it looks like they could do some crochet with that thing and nick the tar out of my hoochy-hoo. But (a) I'm high anxiety, so don't listen to anything I say, and (b) I'll never know because after that there's so much chaos in that little tunnel that a few knitting nicks wouldn't matter anyway. And besides, manually breaking your water never hurts – maybe pinches a bit if you don't have the numb-juice going, but other than that, eh.

Bleeding: Why, *why* do doctors not make it crystal clear that bleeding can signal the onset of dilation? If you're close to your due date and start bleeding, it's time, honey! With all the books we devour and as much as we hound our doctors for information, you'd think this point would be driven home. But with all the well-educated women I know who haven't a clue (including me), this is obviously an overlooked factoid. The night before my scheduled induction with my first baby, I had actually been "pre-induced" with a little pill they stick up your cervix to ripen things up. They sent me home and told me to come in at seven the next morning. Nothing about bleeding. Nooo, no. So at four in the morning, I'm in the bathtub trying to ease the contractions (the little pill worked, by golly!) until it was time to leave, and then...blood! There's blood! Surely this means the kid's going to fall out any second!

Somebody please hold my hand and give me a valium – or at least tell me what's going to happen!! Little did Captain Pansy here know, when you dilate, your cervix stretches and you can bleed. Hello! Just a little detail there! All I knew was that bleeding was a No-No, as in "you are four months pregnant and should not be bleeding" or "bleeding could be due to placental abruption." Panic, bad, and get me to a hospital. Got that part. But bleeding during labor? Who knew!

Okay, so adding a few years of wisdom to my life, I can see that a normal person would connect the two and think bleeding=labor. How hard is that? You bleed early or you bleed on time; what's the difference? The difference, Mr. Already Knew That Smarty Pants, is that I always assumed bleeding was bad! No bleeding! Go away! And when I start bleeding, no matter if I'm supposed to or not, if I don't *know* I'm supposed to bleed, I DO know I'm supposed to panic. (Sorry, pregnant gibberish.) Bottom line, YES, you can bleed when you dilate. There. If I saved the world of one hysterical mom-to-be, I've done my job. But still tell your doctor right away. I don't care if you DO tell me to calm down, oh ye medical people who never bothered to clue me in. I may not panic, but I am still going to fret until that baby is out and healthy.

Puking & Shaking

Puking: My friend Amy is the Queen of Puke-in-Labor. She pukes and pukes and takes it all in stride, demanding only that her husband take the offensive kidney dish or hospital measuring cup (what are those used for, anyway? Pee?) and flush the contents down the toilet. He dutifully dumps and rinses, dumps and rinses, until she gets tired of gagging on the smell and orders him to wash the damn thing as well. I, on the other hand, spend the entire time holding up her four feet of blond locks so she can yak without messing up the do. By the way, WHY don't you put your hair in a ponytail? Simple little invention, works wonders. Amy, however, has hair so long that if she needs it up, she just ties it in a knot. No kidding, I doubt it even occurs to her to put it up in a band, much less bring one to the hospital to refrain from puking on Rapunzel's mane.

Anyway, here she is, shaking like a leaf and yakking, and the first time around I thought, huh. People throw up during labor? By the second time around, I thought, oop, she's at it again - must be dilating! "Good news, Amy! You're probably (oooh, ooh, hit the kidney dish, not me, please) on the home stretch!"

So keep a little throw-up bucket right where you can reach it. Whether it's reaction to medication (I'm reaching here), the intensity of your body's change, or just plain nausea due to pain or anxiety, I really have no idea. You don't see or hear about it much, but poopin' on the Doc is nothing; you could *puke* all over the Doc — or nurse, or anesthesiologist, or your husband, for that matter. And *that* is harder to clean up. Yowza.

Shake, Shake, Shake: I may not have much experience with yakking, but shaking, oh yeah. I convulse uncontrollably when in labor, just as normal as you please. People rush around getting me blankets and make lame attempts to calm me down, thinking I must be scared shitless if I'm shaking that much. But no. Just shaking. I don't know why. I always attribute it to epidural or pain medication, but I also know my body freaks out under intense labor pain. If you look it up, there is usually some explanation about hormonal rushes or bodily reactions to the transition phase or the last phase of birth…whatever. You'll probably shake. And you'll most likely get pissed off when people scurry around like chickens, because you are so in The Zone that you just need them to shut up and let you labor in peace.

That is One Big Fat Needle! (Epidural)

Do we get the epidural or do we not get the epidural? Do we spend $800 or do we not spend $800? Eeeny meeny miney moe. Girl, you do whatever the heck you want. In all fairness, I do try to labor without the goose juice, but I usually don't get very far. And fear of the needle can hold you back a while. Just know that unless you are prepped and poised and ready to rock and roll, by the time you request it, it may be a good hour before you get it. Heaven knows how much pain you'll be in then. This is good and bad. Good because you'll be in so much pain that you seriously won't care how big the darn thing is or where the heck they're sticking it. Bad because you are in so much pain that whatever the hell they're doing back there, they better do it fast.

Here's what happens: You either lay on your side or sit up with your legs off the side of the bed, back rounded. You can hug a pillow and lean on a person (hubby or a nurse) or put the pillow on an adjustable bedside table and "lay" on it. From there on out it's just breathing deep and trying not to yowl or wiggle during a contraction until the anesthesiologist is finished. The doctor will ask questions throughout to make sure he's poking the right place (don't think about it). You might feel some pinching here and there, but nothing worse than a contraction, and you'll be a happy camper in about five minutes. Then you get to kick back and relax, pushing a little button for more medication as you need it. The machine is programmed to keep you from sucking too much up at once, but you do have to be careful not to get trigger happy. Otherwise you'll be so numb that your bottom half is effectively "dead," and you won't know a push from a flying pink giraffe. So go easy!

I guess we're at the end of the line here, love! We've covered the biggie-topics, so you should be prepared. Now that you're ready for childbirth (Ho!!) the next chapter deals with just a few post-partum issues that might have been glossed over in your pregnancy library. Oooh, how we hate that!

Chapter Nine: Post-Partum Stuff

Honey, you're going to be so tired once the baby arrives. Reading about post-partum issues will just not happen. So here are a few topics that beg mentioning. Stick them in the back of your mind in case they come up. That way you won't be blind-sided and flip out. There is no flipping out with the support of your girlfriends!

Hospital Goodie Bag

I have to take a moment to dish on a few of the fun items in the goodie bag you get as they roll you out of Labor and Delivery.

Blow Up Donut-Thing: Officially called a hemorrhoid pillow, I loved this thing so much that I almost went so far as to name and christen it as one of the family. I carried that baby everywhere – to church and restaurants – with nary an embarrassed bone in my body. Loved it!

Squeeze & Pee: For those of you out of the loop, after you have a baby, you have to squeeze water on your woo-woo while you pee. You'll be stitched and beat up down there, and urine doesn't exactly feel good. So every time you need to pee, you get your handy little bottle, fill it up with warm water, and squirt away with gusto. If you already have kids, be careful they don't take off with it. It's that fun.

Fishnet Panties: I LOVE THESE THINGS!! Throw away, cloth, fishnet-like undies that stretch and love your lumpy post-partum body –uh! Love fest. Not exactly the sexiest things, as you have to stuff an oven mitt sized pad in there, but no matter. These are the things I look forward to the most from the hospital visit. Flowers and gifts are nice, but wrap me up a box of these and stick a bow on it...I'm crying with joy.

Immediate Shocks

Sweating the Bed: Geez Louise, those post-partum sweats! Your body may go into a freaky relief shock and sweat you out of your bed that first post-partum night. If you bring your own pillow from home, put about a thousand towels on it! Yeesh. And forget about your own pajamas. I know you're dying to get out of that hospital gown, but save it for later. You'll be yanking it off, soaking wet, in the middle of the night anyway. Either keep an extra hospital gown handy, or be prepared to strip down and spend the rest of the night naked as a jaybird (save those sexy mesh panties).

Pain and Bleeding: Even if all goes well, you'll be doing the slow-motion walk for several days or a couple weeks. My Poker Mommy Carey said that if her husband so much as sat next to her on the bed, she'd screech in pain. The goodies were so sore that the movement of the mattress sent her reeling. This is a bit extreme, but still teaches a valuable lesson: respect the baby tunnel.

As far as bleeding, expect it to last in some degree for up to six weeks. It may come and go, but should eventually ease up just like a normal period. Yes, it's sucky to have a pad down there for so long, but you could be like one of my friends and think nothing of it since she's never used a tampon in her entire life. She has no clue what it's like to have a non-gushy period. Claiming to be the only woman on the planet who has never had a tampon violate her hooch, she's just peachy with pads. Believe me, I've given her the whole persuasive, instructional talk complete with pictures. However, she's just positive that wayward tampon will be sucked into her cervix and get lost in her guts. No thank you.

Breast Engorgement: You may not believe it humanly possible, but once your milk comes in, you will give Dolly Parton a total run for her money. One friend told me it was literally the 3rd worse day of her life after parental death and heartbreak. Don't freak and fear it's permanent. Those poor dears will be rock hard and painful enough to make you cry serious tears, but it does pass.

In total desperation after my last delivery, I did the whole wrap-your-jugs-in-cabbage business. I forced my sister to peel off the biggest outside leaves and help me slap those veggies over the hurt mongers, then wrap it all up in an ace bandage. The icy-coldness felt great, but other than that, it seemed like a waste of time. Perhaps I was wallowing in too much misery to see the bright side, but it certainly didn't seem to help dissolve any rigidity. In fact, every time I took off the bandage, my boobs were totally stuck in that flat wrapped-up shape. Unyielding, burning hot, and completely freaky. I'm surprised the cabbage didn't actually cook.

Breast Feeding: A common worry, many women think they need to feed the baby immediately after birth. Surprisingly, I've heard that we need to chill. An L&D nurse friend says that God made your body a certain way, and the baby won't starve if he can't nurse right away. She says to trust your body and relax. Your milk will start flowing at some point, and your engorged and painful knockers will soon be squishy and happy. Until then, indulge in the guidance from your post-partum nurse or a lactation consultant. These people are life savers. Just be prepared for some none-too-shy booby grabbing. They go at it with gusto.

Keep an open mind with breast feeding, because it doesn't always run smoothly. One of the problems can be inverted or flat nipples. You'd think with mongo size Gs the darn things would work, but no - flat nipples. These means Jr. can't latch on. Even if you have great nipples, the baby could still have trouble latching. One of my friends was a total milk machine, but for some reason, neither of her kids could latch on. She tried all the professional advice she could get her hands on, but nothing worked. Sometimes it's pump or bust, ladies. Sadness is bound to overwhelm you, but keep the big picture in mind. Any way you can get your milk into your pooh bear is fine. Seven hellish months of pump joy, here we come!

Pumping: Worth it, but SO time consuming. It's almost like having twins, by the time you pump and then wash the equipment. Take it from the girlfriends: get multiple sets of tubes and cups so you're not washing them every four hours. And buy a pump *before* baby comes so you're not sitting there engorged and drippy during the sales pitch. Ouch!

I must also take a moment to warn you what it looks like to pump. Picture a boob-shaped funnel on your girls and nipples being sucked forward about two feet. I cover my eyes and run every time my friend Amy breaks the damn thing out. Oh man! Not that again! Shield my delicate eyes! Amy is a bumble bee and never actually sits to do anything. So not only is she unnaturally still for 20 minutes a pop, but I have to act composed and calm while it looks like her boobs will surely be vacuumed and torn from her body. On the rational side, she would absolutely tell you I'm a drama queen and pansy, and to ignore my exaggeration and fits of despair. So listen to her and not me. I never breast fed a day in my life, so what do I know? Yes, it's a bit weird at first, but I'm sure you'll deal just fine.

Dumpy body: You know, some us feel kind of mother-nature-y attractive while preggo. Then the baby flops out and eek! We're just a blob. Immediately after birth you're so happy to have that huge bump gone that you think the belly looks positively fab. But wait. Upon closer inspection, the ol' skin is so stretched and mutilated that it ends up looking like a deflated, wrinkly balloon. Mine was even eight shades of brown last time. I begged my dermatologist to help, but she didn't have much optimism. She knew it was simply a time-thing. Over the course of days and weeks, it slowly reshapes, but the process is lumpy and depressing. You'll still need your preggy clothes and undies (cuss worthy). But hang in there, girl! It does get better. It's just sluggish, and one more thing to cry about.

Getting Some Sleep: Headline! *Don't feel guilty for using the nursery at the hospital!!* Seriously ladies, you'll have just been through the ringer. I know you'll be dying to spend every precious moment with your new bundle, but if you can't recover, you can't be a good mommy. It's perfectly okay to let the baby sleep in the nursery so you can catch some much needed zzz's. We promise not to brand you unworthy!

Once you get home, make hubby help and accept all other offers for sitting, housecleaning, food prep – the works. It doesn't make you a bad mom. It makes you a smart mom! You'll be in a 24-hour take-care-of-baby stupor, and must allow yourself time to recover and sleep. Don't try to be a super hero and do it all yourself. After birth, your body goes into some sort of hormone high for about a week. This silly delusion makes you think you're totally rockin' with sleep and mommy-duties. Then about 7-10 days in, it hits like a brick. *"SHIT, I am freaking going psycho if I don't get some help!!"* Trust your girlfriends. Take any help, at any time!

Co-Sleeping: If you want to co-sleep, great. But for the love of Pete, buy a bedside co-sleeper. My friend Kristi kept her son in their bed until, well...okay, he's still in their bed. Although she's never rolled over on the kid, she also didn't get any real sleep for the first year. She stayed half-awake for fear of smothering him. Bad, bad, bad idea. Pregnant again, she's adamant that baby #2 is getting a bedside co-sleeper!

Spouse Issues

A Little Help? Listen up, ladies! Don't expect hubby to notice and do as much as you want automatically - or even after severe nagging. Boys will be boys, and husbands can be oblivious. (Is this news?) They don't see dirt, they're happy living off cold pizza, and if they smell a poopy diaper, the only thing that occurs to them is to holler at you to fix it. With baby #1, you can't possibly anticipate all the areas you'll want his help, but at least have a dialogue about it before birth. Something along the lines of "You'll need to get off your ass and help me when I start screaming."

Do NOT Talk About Sex or You Shall Die!! Can hubby annoy us anymore than asking the doc four times in one visit how soon you can have sex? Uh! In your thoroughly embarrassed and irritated mind, every time he asks, the time frame gets longer - although it's hard to lengthen "NEVER AGAIN YOU CRAZY PERSON!!"

Honey, it's bad enough that he has to wait for sex after birth. If you additionally shut down the shop in the last weeks (or months) of your gestating process, hubster will be all over you for a re-open date. He can't actually see any damage, so what's it to him? He's forgotten all about seeing your goodies stretched to bloody oblivion, and it's obviously had no bearing on your sex appeal. We can shake our heads in wonder, but he'll never understand that we need a couple of months to appreciate his continued desire.

What? No Love Fest? Yes, we're ecstatic to have baby finally arrive. But why must hubby wonder why we're not a blissful Buddha-like new mom? Hmmm, maybe lack of sleep, hormones, and general soreness??? Oh, the pain of it all! When you finally do get a few glorious minutes alone in the shower, in pops hubby with the naked baby. Apparently his perfect family-with-a-new-baby image is straight out of an old Lever 2000 ad, showing the whole family sudsing its collective 6000 parts. My friend Julie's huband tried this on her, and she about tore his eyes out. (Poor, clueless, starry-eyed guy.) Julie told him in no uncertain terms (i.e., screamed like a banshee) that if he EVER dared interrupt her shower again, that would be grounds for divorce. Not to mention that wet babies are crazy slippery and shouldn't be held in a shower. Shouldn't any responsible father automatically know that? This dude certainly should, since Julie had been spending every second of the day worrying about keeping the little lovedoodle breathing! But who cares about details?

Loss of Private Time and Space

Maybe this doesn't sound like a big deal. After all, who wouldn't want to hold a cuddly new baby? And don't they sleep for 16 hours a day anyway? Wrong! This is huge. After the baby comes it can feel like you have someone hanging on you or demanding something every second of the day. If you're pumping, it can be like this: feed the baby, clean the baby, get the baby to sleep, pump, clean the darn pump, try to fit in one chore so your house isn't making you completely mad, then repeat ad nauseum. You may be holding in pee for hours, too busy to go (I'm big on no time to pee). When you finally make it to the toilet, you're miraculously dropping drawers, peeing, and wiping with one hand while holding the crying baby in the other.

Meanwhile, you're starving and scarfing down scraps of cracker or leftover garlic rolls while feeding the kiddo seemingly nonstop. Your clothes get covered in stale breast milk, spit up, and worse (projectile poop, anyone?). So in addition to feeling like a badly-molded lump of flesh, you stink. You won't get to shower for an unknown number of hours. If dear old hubby comes in right then saying he's thinking about catching a movie, it can make you cranky. If he comes in complaining that the baby's getting all the attention and he needs some too, watch out.

Not Feeling Like You're Supposed to Be Feeling

Bonding: You may not feel an overwhelming tidal wave of love the second you set eyes on your little one. If you don't, you may feel guilty or even panic-stricken. Are you ever going to love the poor little guy? Are you going to be a terrible, disconnected mother? Is the kid going to be in therapy for life? Even second-time moms say they didn't instantly feel the same about a new baby as they did about their first born, resulting in the same kinds of worries. It took me weeks to bond with my second kid – and heaven knows why, because she was perfect.

Don't get me wrong. Of course we love our babies from conception. My friend Melanie said that her husband once forgot she was pregnant (bad enough!) and pushed off against her tummy getting up from the sofa. The mommy brain and hormones went crazy at the slight chance he could've smooshed the bambino. She'd never been so instantly and intensely angry in her life. Four years later, she still sees red thinking about it. But fast forward (rewind?) to birth. She didn't know exactly what she was feeling when little Austin opened those peepers and looked at her. Mostly, she felt awkward and fake, like she was just a pretend mom. It takes a while to get used to motherhood. The warm fuzzies come soon enough, but, until they overwhelm the weirdness, you're a tad worried about being Mummy Dearest. Of course, six months down the road, you'll turn to goo just thinking about your sweet angel. The best little buggeroo in the whole world!

Baby Blues: For your standard old blues, while it may not be full blown depression, it's still no bowl of cherries. Between hormones and lack of sleep, the honeymoon is definitely over. It's not quite like pregnancy crying, where nothing in particular can set you off, but you can still boohoo at the drop of a hat. This is just more of a gradual, beaten down kind of weeping. You're exhausted, your nipples are killing you, there's never anything good to eat, and the baby is a constant lovable time suck. Your own needs are shoved to the back of the priority list. WAY back. As in, you only exist to serve. It's a bit depressing! One of my friends said she was just plain angry for a full year.

There's also the possibility of full blown depression. I was on medication for post-partum depression (PPD) for nine months after the birth of my first kid. To this day, I still think it was exhaustion that made me psychotic, but who knows. I couldn't sleep due to horrific nightmares (as in, demons were trying to wrench my newborn out of my hands) and couldn't let go enough to trust my husband with our daughter's care. He was awesome – took to parenting like a duck to water, but I had to be stupid and refuse control. I never wanted her out of my sight, making sure she continued to breathe and had every infinitesimal need met. It was a prescription for disaster, my friend. I finally lacked the will to make it out of bed one day, and we knew things had to change.

Happy enough, I did end up getting off the meds without difficulty. Given my history, the doctor wanted to put me on meds immediately after the birth of baby #2, but I refused. Instead, I let my husband take a big chunk of the work and I got enough rest. (Retrospectively, how insanely brainless do you have to be to refuse fabulous help from your mate? Uh! What a nincompoop!) Sure enough, I was fine. No depression. This is not to say that all PPD is due to lack of sleep. Sometimes brain chemistry gets out of whack no matter what you do. Just keep an open dialogue with your caregiver and do NOT be embarrassed to discuss your post-partum blues. They cannot help you if you don't communicate. If it's regular old blues, they should provide encouragement on what to expect and ways to get through it. But if it's truly depression, you will need the help of a trusted doctor to get you through.

Anxiety Over Life Changes: If you're ending or postponing a career to stay at home, there's a whole set of changes that can be hard to cope with. My friend Melanie is a lawyer and was used to helping close multi-million dollar deals. Gray-haired men in suits would actually listen to her. The hours were long and stressful, but she spent all day in a nice, quiet office fantasizing about being home with her darling newborn. She imagined all the free time she would have to get in shape, take up some old hobbies, and relax with the hubby. (Foolish girl.)

Zoom ahead to post-partum and she suddenly found herself at home, with nothing as she expected. Her most brainy tasks were changing diapers and trying to figure out WHY ON EARTH the kiddo was crying. Yes, she's a lawyerly nerd, but her brain literally hurt from the change in gears. Meanwhile her every move was second-guessed by various friends and family members. (And forget being listened to by gray-haired men - there's apparently some strange suburb rules about talking to men/husbands.) So in addition to the "OMG, I have a baby, what have I done?" question, she was contending with "OMG, I quit my job, what have I done?" In over her head, there was a wee panic attack in the works.

My dear, this will hit you, and you will overcome. No, it's not intellectually stimulating to deal with milk and diapers all day. But give me any old professional big-wig and I'll turn him into a ball of mush in no time flat. They would NEVER be able to keep up with our noble and arduous baby-care schedule. The selfless work of newborn care may seem insignificant to the brainiacs of the world, but I bet they cried a few tears as a child and ran to their Mommy for comfort. Hrumph! I ask you, who's the most important person in the world? The bigwig, or the bigwig's Mommy?

Over and Out

Girl, there is so much more I could write about, but I'm freaking tired. Aside from the fact that I absolutely cannot navigate my mongo belly to reach the keyboard one minute longer, I am DYING to sleep for the next two weeks until my little visitor shows up. I'm so cranky, miserable, and exhausted that there is not one sympathetic bone left in my body. Amy has called me three times today, leaving messages that she has simply GOT to go to the grocery store and her toddler is driving her nuts. Can I please, please, watch her for an hour?? Please?

Amy doesn't usually get this desperate, so I know it's bad. But I still ignored the phone (can't even muster the energy to answer it), only to have her show up on my doorstep, harried beyond belief, practically dragging this poor kid by her armpits. Did I do the best friend thing and lovingly sweep little Miss Lily into my house to join my crew? Nope. Pack that kid back up in your car, because I've got a date with the couch. I'll ask for forgiveness later.

I'm gonna go have a baby now, so I'll see you lovely gals on the other side. Much love and best wishes! Moms Rock!

Author's Note

You know, this really was written while pregnant with my third child. But two weeks before delivery I screamed, "I CANNOT write anymore!!" So I hit save, flopped on the couch, and tried not to move a muscle until necessary. I had a three-year-old and a four-year-old, so it wasn't easy, but you stock the pantry and fridge with fish crackers, turkey slices, and cheese cubes within toddler grabbing range, and you're good to go for a few hours.

Skip ahead a year or two, and I wanted to finish up my toddler books so I could continue to capture the perspective of actually going through toddlerhood as I wrote. Then I went back to work as a speech therapist, and, well, now it's six...years...later. Good news is, I sleep more – although that's quite recent and took an internist to discover a sleep disorder (thank you SO much). On the one hand, it's good to know the reason for your freakish fatigue and general psychosis, but since I refuse medication (that tree-hugger thing again), keeping up with the diet and exercise changes are a chore.

So, while babyhood and toddlerhood are a recent memory, and life is kicking again, feel sure that while writing, I DO feel your pain and hopefully share some insight and misery. We are sisters in preggy-land, bonding away and sharing the love!

As an aside, I'm sure you realize by now that I'm quite outspoken. Please forgive any outlandish indiscretions! While I tried to remain decent enough to keep the cussing and graphics to a non-raunchy level, I simply could not write a boring book, adding to the collective snores of pregnant readers. We need to have some fun.

I hope your reading was happy. Best wishes on your blessed day! I love ya, girl!

About the Author

Michelle Smith is a Speech-Language Pathologist, working with kids from preschool to high school. She lives in Texas, adores her three girls, and enjoys reading, sleeping (woohoo!), and taking care of her enormous Maine Coon cat. This is Michelle's third book behind *Life with Toddlers* and the *Toddler ABC Guide to Discipline*. Her unique perspective and distinct voice allows her to encourage, entertain, and empower caregivers with heart-felt, professional, and realistic advice.

Get in-depth information about how to get the best behavior from your toddler in *Life with Toddlers*!

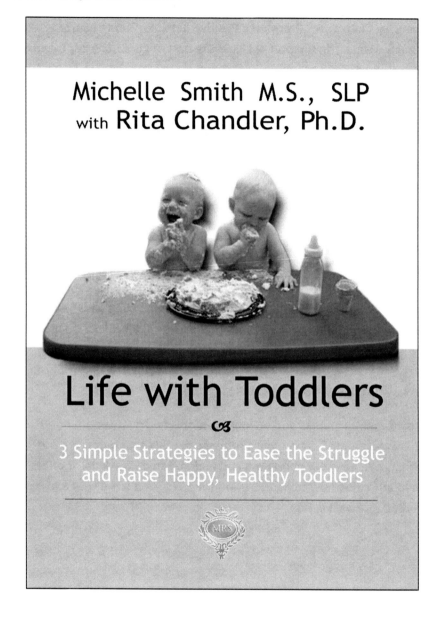

Michelle Smith M.S., SLP
with **Rita Chandler, Ph.D.**

Life with Toddlers
cs
3 Simple Strategies to Ease the Struggle
and Raise Happy, Healthy Toddlers

Reviews for *Life with Toddlers*:

"Funny - Easy to read but packed with lots of good information. Especially Chapter 4: "Promoting Positive Behavior" and Chapter 8: "Taming Tigers". In Chapter 4, I liked the part of giving choices to your toddler instead of just issuing orders and frustrating them to anger and tears. In Chapter 8: "Taming Tigers" - "But I Waaannnttt It" (How many times have you heard this in Walmart??) - I think these words of wisdom should be posted in the store's lobby. - Loved this book!" - **Sandi J.**

"This book is like having a hundred frank what-am-I-supposed-to-do-now girlfriend talks handy on your shelf. Throughout, the advice is easy to remember and use, I think even when your little one is screaming his head off. The book helped me understand my son's behavior, making it loads easier to avoid frazzled-mom-emergency mode. I tried some tips right after reading them and had my child following instructions without whining, hooray! I especially appreciated the section on what you can (and shouldn't) do when it's someone else's child acting badly. My mommy friends and I have debated that touchy subject sooooo much, so it's super helpful to have the author's insight. As a bonus, the author's friendly, no-nonsense style had me giggling (and snorting) all the way through the book." - **Leslie**.

"Most parenting books end up making moms feel guilty about not being the "perfect mom". This book addresses the fact that moms are not perfect. We have our good days and bad and so do our kids. It offers sound advice on how to handle real situations - and it is a very easy and fun read." - **Pickle & Bug**.

If you have a friend or relative that needs the boiled down, fast version of Life with Toddlers, then the Toddler ABC Guide to Discipline is the answer.

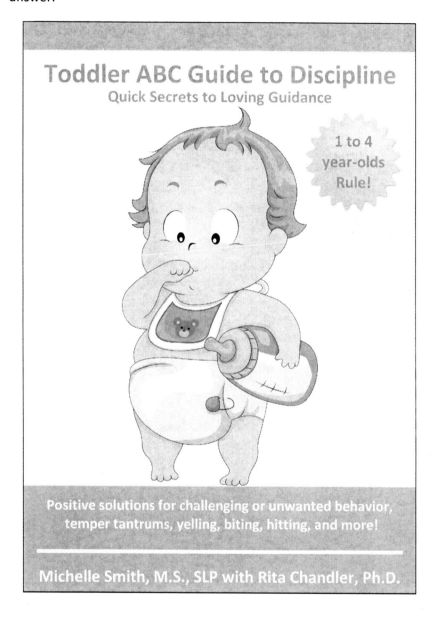

Toddler ABC Guide to Discipline
Quick Secrets to Loving Guidance

1 to 4 year-olds Rule!

Positive solutions for challenging or unwanted behavior, temper tantrums, yelling, biting, hitting, and more!

Michelle Smith, M.S., SLP with Rita Chandler, Ph.D.

Reviews for the *Toddler ABC Guide to Discipline*:

"I pick this book up and could immediately relate to the issues the author talks about. As a home-school dad I am always on the look out for quality materials that can greatly benefit and inspire both the parent and the child. Too many times I have heard parents ask "When is the best time to start positive instruction?". The answer is now, and this book is your road map." - **E.T. Pate**.

"This book is a quick and easy read for a busy mom. It gets the point across in a entertaining and informative way. It certainly made me rethink how to handle bad behavior. I loved the author's techniques because they are positive, very passive and they really work!!! I would highly recommend this book to all mom's and dad's." - **Sandy M**.

CPSIA information can be obtained at www.ICGtesting.com
Printed in the USA
LVOW121155050212

267147LV00015B/122/P